SpringerBriefs in Computer Science

SpringerBriefs present concise summaries of cutting-edge research and practical applications across a wide spectrum of fields. Featuring compact volumes of 50 to 125 pages, the series covers a range of content from professional to academic.

Typical topics might include:

- A timely report of state-of-the art analytical techniques
- A bridge between new research results, as published in journal articles, and a contextual literature review
- A snapshot of a hot or emerging topic
- An in-depth case study or clinical example
- A presentation of core concepts that students must understand in order to make independent contributions

Briefs allow authors to present their ideas and readers to absorb them with minimal time investment. Briefs will be published as part of Springer's eBook collection, with millions of users worldwide. In addition, Briefs will be available for individual print and electronic purchase. Briefs are characterized by fast, global electronic dissemination, standard publishing contracts, easy-to-use manuscript preparation and formatting guidelines, and expedited production schedules. We aim for publication 8–12 weeks after acceptance. Both solicited and unsolicited manuscripts are considered for publication in this series.

**Indexing: This series is indexed in Scopus, Ei-Compendex, and zbMATH **

Cristian Axenie · Roman Bauer ·
Oliver López Corona · Jeffrey West

Applied Antifragility in Natural Systems

From Principles to Applications

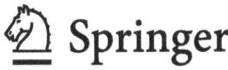

Cristian Axenie
Department of Computer Science
and Center for Artificial Intelligence
Technische Hochschule Nürnberg Georg
Simon Ohm
Nuremberg, Bayern, Germany

Oliver López Corona
Instituto de Investigaciones en Matemáticas
Aplicadas y en Sistemas (IIMAS)
Universidad Nacional Autónoma de México
Mexico City, Mexico

Roman Bauer
Computer Science Research Centre
University of Surrey
Surrey, UK

Jeffrey West
Integrated Mathematical Oncology
Moffitt Cancer Center
Tampa, FL, USA

ISSN 2191-5768   ISSN 2191-5776 (electronic)
SpringerBriefs in Computer Science
ISBN 978-3-031-90390-8   ISBN 978-3-031-90391-5 (eBook)
https://doi.org/10.1007/978-3-031-90391-5

© The Editor(s) (if applicable) and The Author(s), under exclusive license to Springer Nature Switzerland AG 2025

This work is subject to copyright. All rights are solely and exclusively licensed by the Publisher, whether the whole or part of the material is concerned, specifically the rights of translation, reprinting, reuse of illustrations, recitation, broadcasting, reproduction on microfilms or in any other physical way, and transmission or information storage and retrieval, electronic adaptation, computer software, or by similar or dissimilar methodology now known or hereafter developed.
The use of general descriptive names, registered names, trademarks, service marks, etc. in this publication does not imply, even in the absence of a specific statement, that such names are exempt from the relevant protective laws and regulations and therefore free for general use.
The publisher, the authors and the editors are safe to assume that the advice and information in this book are believed to be true and accurate at the date of publication. Neither the publisher nor the authors or the editors give a warranty, expressed or implied, with respect to the material contained herein or for any errors or omissions that may have been made. The publisher remains neutral with regard to jurisdictional claims in published maps and institutional affiliations.

This Springer imprint is published by the registered company Springer Nature Switzerland AG
The registered company address is: Gewerbestrasse 11, 6330 Cham, Switzerland

If disposing of this product, please recycle the paper.

This book is about and for nature's systems, where antifragility offers the recipe to turn uncertainty, evolution's random mutations, and volatility into lasting advantages.

Foreword

What is Antifragility?

Abstract
Antifragility is a unifying mathematical modeling framework transferring properties from the functional domain of dose-response into the probabilistic one in distribution of outcomes, and vice versa.

Consider the following seemingly disconnected or loosely connected classes of natural and human phenomena:

Class 1 *Upregulation: Effects related to benefiting from stressors.* These include hormesis and hypertrophy in medicine, post-traumatic growth in psychology, tumor resistance in oncology, hydra-like outcomes in mythology, as well as popular beliefs about rebounds from adversity.

Class 2 *Philostochasticity: Effects related to benefiting from variance and dispersion.* These include stochastic resonance in physics and signal processing, intermittent fasting and variable dosing in medicine, "long" volatility in finance. Evolutionary processes require a certain dose of noise, variance, or replication error to satisfy a diversity of outcomes, with the hope that some of the resulting offspring will be more adapted to the environment.

Class 3 *Scaling: Effects related to allometry.* These include optimal size of animals, cities, and corporations, the fragility induced by an increase in size (stochastic diseconomies of scale), the behavior of biological entities at different scales.

Now note the property of items with opposite qualitative attributes.

Class 4 *Fragility: Effects related to breaking or rupturing under shocks and stressors at some intensity.*

Class 5 *Short volatility: harm by dispersion of outcomes and second-order effects at some window or time interval.* For example eating continuously might be harmful, but intermittently can only benefit at some time window (while a daily or alternate day occurrence may help, a monthly one can be deadly).

Class 6 *Effects linked to hazards associated with the passage of time*: it includes decay from memoryless shocks, aging, ruin probabilities, and absorbing barriers.

The idea behind antifragility isn't a descriptive approach to these attributes, nor an uncovering of these well observed phenomena, but a unifying mathematical modeling framework integrating all these classes, and, centrally **transferring properties from the functional domain of dose-response into the probabilistic one**.

Let y be the response, $y = f(x)$ a function of X a random (or deterministic) variable; we are concerned with $f(x)$; and the nonlinearity of f is determinant in altering the statistical properties of x. Functions in most applications are piecewise convex or concave, giving a rich set of responses—in general, the more nonlinear f, the more its outcomes will be divorced from the statistical properties of X.

Critically, we may not observe the full properties of X, owing to statistical incompleteness, idiosyncratic behavior, and sample insufficiency; but we can certainly assess the behavior of f via perturbation methods, in the body and the tails of the distribution. We can even sometimes influence the function, a method dubbed "convexification" or "tail clipping" applicable in finance. The idea of contracts is to eliminate, share, or transfer parts of the distribution, which alters the probability distribution of f.

The entire concept is based on a definition of fragility, which in [1, 2] is grounded in the following property. Fragility, for probabilistic reasons, must be accompanied by an accelerated response to harm, as the cumulative effect of regular, high-frequency events must be smaller in effect than those stemming from the tails of the distribution. This is a selection effect akin to the survivorship bias: being linear to harm would necessarily break the object under an ordinary intensity of stressors; what has survived must be nonlinear, having a milder response in the body of the distribution and a stronger one away from the center. Estimating the effects of tail risk resides in the nonlinearity of the response with respect to tail events [4], thus facilitating robust stress testing by focusing on acceleration rather than just magnitude.

Further, an accelerating (super-linear) response to negative stressors (as well as the passage of time) and a decelerating (sub-linear) response to positive outcomes portend fragility; the reverse situations represent antifragility, limited of course to a specific range of variations and a certain time window.

One can be fragile outside a range of variation, anti-fragile inside (though not the opposite). For antifragility is not the mirror opposite of fragility. Irreparable breaking is an absorbing barrier, which stops the unit at the point of non-recoverable ruin. The antifragile does not get absorbed in a similar manner; the asymmetry generates analytical difficulties. We also note that fragility and antifragility are associated with a *specific* source of variation. Natural systems, particularly biological ones, are universally nonlinear in their responses (sometimes extreme where the effect changes in sign, as reflected by the expression "the dose makes the poison"); hence, they lend themselves to analyses translating from the functional to the probabilistic and reciprocally, inviting a spate of medical applications [3].

One area of research with great potential can exploit the property that the transfer from the functional to the probabilistic can also take place in the reverse direction. One such prospective medical application is figuring out the frequency of past famines or shortages in food groups (say, protein) in the habitat from which a certain human groups was adapted. To take a simple application: it can consist in assessing how the intermittence of feeding increases or decreases insulin sensitivity or some other target metric, or assessing the optimal frequency of deprivation for autophagy. The method can also shed some light on the process of aging from the mismatch between lifestyle and ancestral statistical properties, in addition to the root of many diseases stemming from the deprivation of stressors.

We note that both what we call "technical systems", that is, largely manmade and engineered, and the "natural" ones, that is, largely biological, share the same properties; this likely stems from their partaking of the same attributes of nonlinearities, particularly when looked upon dynamically rather than by using comparative statics.

This volume explores the rich sets of outcomes that result from the investigation of the properties of the function $f(.)$ in a variety of domains.

Atlanta, GA, USA   Nassim Nicholas Taleb

References

1. N. N. Taleb, *Antifragile: things that gain from disorder*. Random House and Penguin, 2012.
2. N. N. Taleb and R. Douady, "Mathematical definition, mapping, and detection of (anti)fragility," *Quantitative Finance*, 2013.
3. Taleb, N. N., & West, J. (2023). Working with convex responses: Antifragility from finance to oncology. *Entropy*, 25(2), 343.
4. N. N. Taleb., Canetti, E., Kinda, T., Loukoianova, E. & Schmieder, C. A new heuristic measure of fragility and tail risks: application to stress testing. *International Monetary Fund*, 2013.

Preface

This book's idea and goal are nothing more than a scientific tour-de-force that started just 10 years after Nassim Taleb first introduced antifragility. Pushing the boundaries of the conceptual work Taleb carried in his book, we go interdisciplinary. Using dynamical systems as a common language, we analyzed, developed, and collected insights on how natural (dynamical) systems can turn antifragile. As Taleb described in the foreword to this work, a central goal is to provide a mathematical framework to translate intrinsic properties within the function domain into the probabilistic domain. To describe naturally occurring phenomena, we have organized the chapters into increasingly complex scales: ecological, evolutionary, and interventional antifragility, respectively. We are developing and building cross-domain "recipes" to detect and quantify antifragility in natural systems. In a rather engineered approach, we propose a versatile framework for the analysis and design of antifragile systems, covering biomedicine, biology, ecology, and neuroscience. We hope that this initial effort will motivate scientists to start considering antifragility as a viable approach to studying the role of variation, perturbations, and noise across a wide range of phenomena.

Nuremberg, Germany	Cristian Axenie
Surrey, UK	Roman Bauer
Mexico City, Mexico	Oliver López Corona
Tampa, FL, USA	Jeffrey West
February 2025	

Acknowledgements The Applied Antifragility Research Group would like to thank Mr. Nassim Nicholas Taleb for formalizing the concept of antifragility and for the multiple interactions we had that helped us to refine the applied dimension of this framework. The group's mission is to build a foundational knowledge base by applying antifragile system design, analysis, and development across domains. We are interested in formalizing principles and an apparatus that turns the basic concept of antifragility into a tool for designing and building closed-loop systems that behave beyond robust in the face of uncertainty, volatility, and stress. We are a very diverse group of researchers from different fields. Such an interdisciplinary constellation allows us to explore applied antifragility through multiple lenses and take various research paths. Our latest research is curated and featured on the group's website at https://www.antifragility.science/.

Competing Interests The authors have no competing interests to declare that are relevant to the content of this manuscript.

Contents

1 Introduction 1
   1.1 Motivation and Definitions 1
   1.2 Ecological Antifragility 1
   1.3 Evolutionary Antifragility 2
   1.4 Interventional Antifragility 2
   1.5 Summary 2
   References 3

2 Ecological Antifragility 5
   2.1 Defining Ecological Antifragility 5
      2.1.1 Convexity in Dose Response 6
      2.1.2 Caveats and Future Considerations 7
   2.2 Ecological Antifragility in Medicine 8
      2.2.1 Current Applications in Medicine 9
   2.3 Ecological Planetary Antifragility 10
      2.3.1 Introduction to Planetary Crisis and Antifragility ... 11
      2.3.2 Theoretical Foundations 12
      2.3.3 Measuring Planetary Antifragility 14
      2.3.4 Remarks 15
   2.4 Neuronal Antifragility 18
      2.4.1 Neural Correlates and Representations of Uncertainty ... 19
      2.4.2 Robustness and Resilience in Neuronal Processing ... 20
      2.4.3 Robust Sensorimotor Control Under Uncertainty ... 21
      2.4.4 Antifragility in Sensorimotor Processing 22
   References 26

3 Evolutionary Antifragility 33
3.1 Defining Evolutionary Antifragility 33
3.2 Probability Convolution for Convex and Concave Functions 33
3.3 Evolutionary Antifragility in Medicine 35
3.3.1 Inferring (Anti)-Fragility from Kaplan-Meier Curves 35
3.3.2 Current Applications in Medicine 37
3.4 Threshold Effects Lead to Antifragility 38
3.5 We Are Not Trees but Forests 39
3.5.1 Evolutionary Implications of the Holobiont Concept 40
3.5.2 The Microbiota-Gut-Brain Axis as a Model for Antifragility 41
3.5.3 Impact of Diet and Lifestyle on Holobiont Antifragility 42
3.5.4 Social Dimension of the Holobiont 44
3.6 Implications for Health and Evolutionary Biology 46
3.7 Evolutionary Creative Destruction Enables Antifragility 48
References 49

4 Interventional Antifragility 55
4.1 Defining Interventional Antifragility 55
4.2 Closed-Loop Antifragility in Tumor-Immune-Drug Dynamics 55
4.2.1 Problem Statement 56
4.2.2 Closed-Loop Interventions in Cancer Therapy 57
4.2.3 Tumor–Immune–Drug Network Model 57
4.2.4 Interventional Antifragility Control 59
4.2.5 State-of-The-Art Control Algorithms in Cancer Therapy 64
4.2.6 Interventional Antifragility in Clinical Practice 70
4.3 Closed-Loop Control of Epilepsy 72
4.3.1 Problem Statement 72
4.3.2 Personalization of Therapeutic Intervention in Epilepsy 73
References 74

5 Conclusions 77
5.1 Ecological (Anti)-Fragility 77
5.2 Evolutionary (Anti)-Fragility 78
5.3 Interventional (Anti)-Fragility 79
References 80

Chapter 1
Introduction

Abstract The concept of antifragility pertains to the benefit derived from the variability inherent to a dynamical system, particularly in response to perturbations. This chapter briefly introduces the properties of antifragility in natural systems. These will serve as guidelines to detect, analyse, and model antifragile behavior in various natural systems.

1.1 Motivation and Definitions

Antifragility is the concept that a system (or an organism) can derive quantifiable benefit from external volatility. This term has been applied to various applications and carries a precise, mathematical definition. Mathematically, antifragility is defined as a system with a concave payoff function. Here, the payoff function is the function that describes a system's output response to input. The term initially was applied to financial risk analysis, but these mathematical principles were later applied in biology [1], urban planning, socio-economics, risk analysis [3] and more. Previously, we defined three scales of antifragility in natural (biological) systems: ecological, evolutionary, and interventional, as depicted in Fig. 1.1. We briefly review each scale's definitions and some examples here [2].

1.2 Ecological Antifragility

The first scale is ecological antifragility. Ecology describes the relationship between an organism and the changes to its environment. Similarly, ecological antifragility describes the relationship between an organism and volatile environmental perturbations. Ecological antifragility quantifies a system's internal response dynamics without reference to external interactions (e.g., competing species) or intervention (e.g., therapeutic interventions). Typically, these systems are homogeneous and possess a well-characterized payoff function describing the response dynamics.

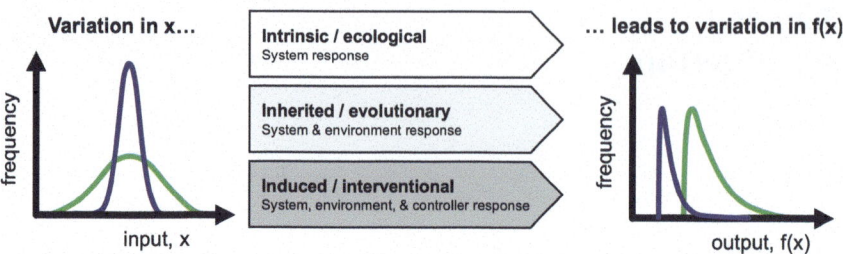

Fig. 1.1 Antifragility-associated terms, defined for technical and natural (biological) systems. Figure reproduced from [2]

1.3 Evolutionary Antifragility

The second scale is evolutionary antifragility. Evolution describes heritable changes in the traits within a heterogeneous population due to changes in its environment, which induce natural selection. Similarly, evolutionary antifragility describes the relationship between a population of individuals and volatile environmental perturbations. Unlike the ecological scale, here we do consider external interactions within the system that modulate the organism's internal response dynamics. Typically, these systems are heterogeneous with a time-dependent or indeterminate payoff function.

1.4 Interventional Antifragility

The final scale is interventional antifragility. Here, we introduce external control or driving signals intended to steer the behavior of a system. Here, a prescribed dynamics is to be attained in the presence of a driving signal additive to the system's dynamics and its uncertainty and perturbations profile.

1.5 Summary

The initial set of definitions allows us to embark on a journey to analyze, model, and design antifragile systems in the realm of natural (dynamical) systems. Please note that we will complement the rather domain-specific modelling and analysis with "recipes" for analysis, quantification, and design of antifragile behaviours.

References

1. Pineda, O., Kim, H. & Gershenson, C. Antifragility of random Boolean networks. *ArXiv Preprint ArXiv:1812.06760* (2018).
2. Axenie, C., López-Corona, O., Makridis, M., Akbarzadeh, M., Saveriano, M., Stancu, A. & West, J. Antifragility in complex dynamical systems. *Npj Complexity*. **1**, 12 (2024).
3. Johnson, J. & Gheorghe, A. Antifragility analysis and measurement framework for systems of systems. *International Journal Of Disaster Risk Science*. **4** pp. 159-168 (2013).

Chapter 2
Ecological Antifragility

Abstract This chapter introduces ecological antifragility as the innate characteristic of a natural dynamic system. It describes the benefit derived from input distribution unevenness, based on the convexity of the response function of the system under uncertainty and volatility. We consider methods for the detection, analysis, and modelling of cancer, ecosystem, and neuronal systems antifragility.

2.1 Defining Ecological Antifragility

Ecological antifragility is defined as the benefit of input distribution unevenness, volatility, or perturbations attributed to the non-linearity of the system's payoff function. Often, a biological system can be well-characterized by a mathematical model describing the relationship between inputs, x, and outputs, $f(x)$. In such cases where perturbing the input increases the resulting output, we use the term antifragility. Ecological antifragility considers the biological system in isolation (without respect to environmental perturbations, evolution by natural selection, or other external interventions) to quantify the response to perturbations. We note that in previous work in physical systems, this scale has been referred to as "intrinsic" antifragility.[1]

We begin by reviewing a formal definition of antifragility and providing several forms of the definition to gain intuition. Broadly, antifragility quantifies the benefit gained from changes to the input distribution. In particular, ecological antifragility describes the scale at which this benefit is derived from the system's intrinsic response. Given a system that is well-characterized by a payoff function, $f(x)$, the benefit (or harm) derived from variation in the input distribution can be quantified directly. Consider the two example functions in Fig. 2.1. Antifragility is closely related to Jensen's Inequality, which compares the expected value of a function to the function evaluated at the expected value [2, 6]. For a convex function $f(x)$, the inequality can be written:

$$\mathbb{E}(f(x)) > f(\mathbb{E}(x)). \tag{2.1}$$

---

[1] We acknowledge the contribution of Mrs Elvia Ramírez-Carrillo from Universidad Nacional Autónoma de México in writing this chapter.

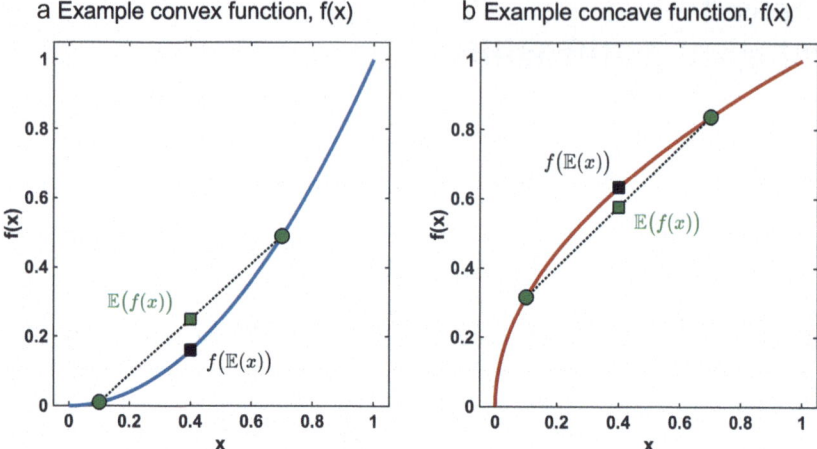

Fig. 2.1 a Example convex function, where $f(x) = x^2$. Response to a high and low dose (e.g. eqn. (2.4)) where $x = 0.4$ and $\Delta = 0.3$ is shown by green circles and compared to a constant dose of $x = 0.4$ (black square). The average of the high and low dose, $\mathbb{E}(f(x))$ (green square), outperforms the response to the average dose, $f(\mathbb{E}(x))$. **b** Example concave function, where $f(x) = x^{\frac{1}{2}}$, where the opposite conclusion is drawn: $\mathbb{E}(f(x)) < f(\mathbb{E}(x))$

The inequality is determined by the geometric shape of $f(x)$. Conversely, if $f(x)$ is concave the inequality will be flipped:

$$\mathbb{E}(f(x)) < f(\mathbb{E}(x)). \qquad (2.2)$$

It is also possible that the function $f(x)$ is linear, thus exactly equivalent:

$$\mathbb{E}(f(x)) = f(\mathbb{E}(x)). \qquad (2.3)$$

Thus, the payoff function representing a system determines whether input variation can maximize $f(x)$ (antifragile; convex) or minimize $f(x)$ (fragile; concave). We note that $f(x)$ can be defined as a positive (favorable) function of benefit (as it is above) or a negative (harmful) function, which will flip the interpretation of antifragility/fragility without loss of generality.

2.1.1 Convexity in Dose Response

To further gain intuition, consider the example of dose-effect in medicine. We compare the effect of a dose, x, to an alternative dosing schema of 120% x followed by a lower dose of 80% x. If the dose response is convex, we expect:

2.1 Defining Ecological Antifragility

$$\frac{f(x+\Delta) + f(x-\Delta)}{2} > f(x) \qquad (2.4)$$

The left-hand side is the average (indeed, the expectation, $\mathbb{E}(f(x))$) of several dose effects, while the right-hand side is the function evaluated at the average dose, or $f(\mathbb{E}(x))$. This is illustrated in Fig. 2.1a, where the right-hand side is marked with a black square while the left-hand side is marked with a green square, denoting the average of the high and low doses (green circles). If the dose-response is concave, the inequality is flipped, and the black square is above the green square.

This simple example can be extended to weigh the effect of the two uneven doses by the time spent on the dose:

$$\lambda f(x+\Delta) + (1-\lambda) f(x-\Delta) > f(x), \qquad (2.5)$$

where $0 \geq \lambda \geq 1$. Previously, Eq. 2.4 is a special case for $\lambda = 0.5$. Thus, it's straightforward to arrive at the following general definition of antifragility:

$$\sum_i^N \lambda_i f(x_i) > f\left(\sum_i^N \lambda_i x_i\right) \qquad (2.6)$$

where each λ_i value is a weight such that $\lambda_i \in [0, 1]$ and $\sum_i \lambda_i = 1$.

An example is shown in Fig. 2.2a, where we have a set of discrete input values, $\mathbf{X} = (x_1, x_2, \ldots, x_N)$ with corresponding weights $\Lambda = (\lambda_1, \lambda_2, \ldots, \lambda_N)$. Next, we show the distribution of values of $\lambda_i x(x_i)$ in Fig. 2.2b, c for the convex and concave functions in the previous figure, respectively. We make several important observations. Firstly, again, the sign of Jensen's inequality is determined by the curvature (convex or concave) of the function $f(x)$. Secondly, while the input distribution of weights, λ, is normally distributed, the output distributions are skewed with a tail to the right (convex) or left (concave). These tails drive the $\mathbb{E}(f(x))$ toward the tail (shown in green dashed line) when compared with the $f(\mathbb{E}(x))$ (black dashed line).

2.1.2 Caveats and Future Considerations

It's important to note that each of these formulations implicitly assumes that the effect of each input (e.g. each dose administered) is independent and additive. This analysis motivates moving from a discrete distribution of weights to a continuous distribution, which we will discuss in the next chapter. Discrete λ_i will be replaced by continuous probability distribution functions, and convolutional methods are employed. In this chapter, we typically deal with cases where the payoff function, $f(x)$, is well known and any external disturbances or environmental signals which alter $f(x)$ are negligible. Without loss of generality, $f(x)$ can describe either benefit or harm to a system,

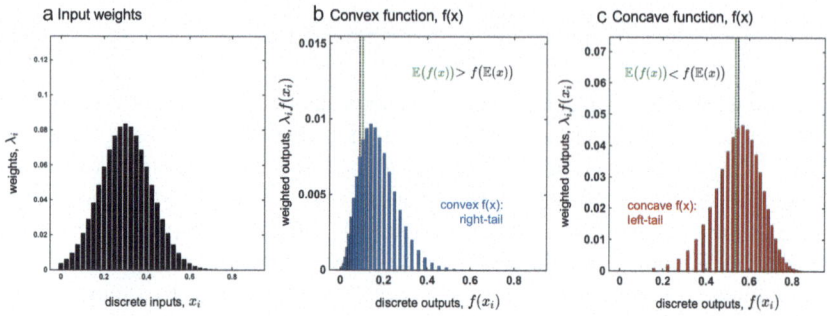

Fig. 2.2 **a** Consider a discrete random variable, **X**, which has discrete values $\mathbf{X} = (x_1, x_2, \ldots, x_N)$ and corresponding weights $\Lambda = (\lambda_1, \lambda_2, \ldots, \lambda_N)$. Input weights are normally distributed with mean $\mu = 0.3$ and standard deviation $\sigma = 0.12$. **b, c** We plot the distribution of weighted outcomes, $\lambda_i f(x_i)$ for the corresponding convex (**b**) and concave (**c**) functions in Fig. 2.1. For convex functions (**b**), the right tail drives the mean of the outcome distribution up so that $\mathbb{E}(f(x)) > f(\mathbb{E}(x))$. For concave functions, the left tail drives the mean down, so that $\mathbb{E}(f(x)) < f(\mathbb{E}(x))$

and thus we can flip the inequality in our definition of antifragility to maximize benefit or minimize harm, respectively.

2.2 Ecological Antifragility in Medicine

Next, we illustrate a simple example of antifragility applied to medicine. Consider a population of tumor cells under treatment with initial size n_0 and growth rate $\gamma(x)$ the final size, n, is given by:

$$n(T) = n_0 \exp(\gamma(x)T), \tag{2.7}$$

where $\gamma(x)$ is the rate of growth of the tumor under treatment with dose x over a time interval of T. The quantity within the parenthesis is known as the log-kill effect, which we denote by the parameter $\beta(x) = \gamma(x)T$. Thus, the effect of multiple doses can be predicted via a summation of the log-kill effect.

$$n = n_0 \exp\left(\beta(x) + \beta(x)\right). \tag{2.8}$$

Next, we assess the effect of variation in the input dose, x, by comparing an even (non-volatile) dosing scheme to an uneven (volatile) dosing scheme. Consider a cycle of treatment:

$$\text{Treatment Cycle} = \{\bar{x} + \Delta, \quad \bar{x} - \Delta\} \tag{2.9}$$

2.2 Ecological Antifragility in Medicine

where $\bar{x}$ represents the dosing schedule's mean dose value and Δ represents the dosing schedule's variance. In this way, all treatment schedules have identical dose mean, enabling us to compare second-order effects that are due to alterations in variance only. We term a dosing schedule "even" if there is no variance ($\Delta = 0$) or "uneven" if the variance is non-zero ($\Delta > 0$).

$$n_{\text{even}} = n_0 \exp\left(\beta(x) + \beta(x)\right)$$
$$n_{\text{uneven}} = n_0 \exp\left(\beta(x + \Delta) + \beta(x - \Delta)\right)$$

As mentioned above, the definition of antifragility (e.g. Eq. (2.4)) requires that the effect of each input is additive and independent. The dose-dependent log-kill rate, $\beta(x)$, satisfies both conditions. Thus, it is useful to define a metric of fragility, F, to compare the log-kill rate of a tumor under even ($\sigma = 0$) dosing or under uneven ($\sigma > 0$) dosing:

$$F(x, \Delta) = \beta(x + \Delta) + \beta(x - \Delta) - 2\beta(x). \tag{2.10}$$

If uneven treatment protocols result in maximizing tumor regression, then it will result in $F < 0$, and we term this situation antifragile. Conversely, if even dosing protocols result in maximizing tumor regression, $F > 0$, it is fragile.

Rearranging some terms, it's straightforward to show the following relation:

$$F = \ln\left(\frac{n_{\text{uneven}}}{n_{\text{even}}}\right) \tag{2.11}$$

Or, more conveniently:

$$n_{\text{uneven}} = n_{\text{even}} \exp(F). \tag{2.12}$$

Therefore, fragility, F, is interpreted as the log-kill gain (or loss) of switching to an uneven treatment schedule, compared to baseline even dosing. Patients will benefit (i.e. maximizing tumor kill) by switching to an uneven dosing protocol when $F < 0$. The appropriate measure of convexity is the exponential growth rate of tumors as a function of dose delivered, $\beta(x)$, and therefore precise characterization of the convexity (or concavity) of this function is warranted. Examples are shown in Fig. 2.3.

2.2.1 Current Applications in Medicine

The most common treatment paradigm in cancer treatment is the maximum-tolerable-dose (MTD) paradigm, where the goal is to escalate the dose to the maximum extent possible while managing toxic side effects [3]. This is equivalent to maximizing "first-order effects" by increasing the cumulative dose by dose-dense chemotherapy [4].

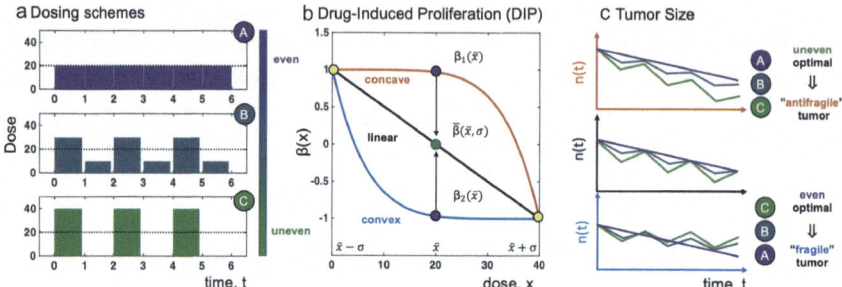

Fig. 2.3 Dose response convexity predicts optimal treatment schedule. **a** Schematics of even (purple) and uneven (green) treatment schedules with the same cumulative dose delivered. **b** Examples of dose-response curves with differing convexity. The green dot indicates the difference between the average $\beta(x)$ for two doses versus the $\beta(x)$ at the average dose delivered. C Predicted tumor size based on each dose-response curve. When the dose-response is concave, more tumor is eliminated by uneven treatment cycles, so the tumor is antifragile. Conversely, if the dose-response is convex, then even treatment cycles are preferable, and the tumor is fragile. Figure adapted from Ref. [13]

Alternative treatment strategies, such as frequent low dosing using metronomic therapy, still implicitly optimize the first-order effect of a cumulative dose while ignoring any second-order effects that result from changing the variance of dosing [6].

For example, second-order effects can be manipulated through the use of high/low dosing [4, 7]. The clinical feasibility of increasing a dose (when paired with a subsequent lower dose) has been demonstrated in intermittent high dosing of tyrosine kinase inhibitors (TKI) in HER2- breast cancer [8], intermittent ribociclib dosing in ER+ breast [9], or intermittent erlotinib in EGFR-mutant lung cancer [10]. This dosing approach, also known as uneven dosing, is a promising strategy when the dose-response is convex (see Fig. 2.1). Another justification for increasing the dose may be rooted in the partial sensitivity of resistant subpopulations within a tumor: a higher dose is required for an effective response against resistance mechanisms. Mathematical modeling is an ideal tool to build an in-silico framework used for making predictions based on clinical data [11, 12]. Other recent mathematical approaches to second-order effects in medicine include investigations into threshold effects [4], the influence of pharmacokinetics on uneven dosing protocols [13], and the influence of cell-cell interactions in heterogeneous tumors [14]. These approaches are typically limited to fixed, periodic treatment schedules, but we will discuss adaptive, non-fixed approaches to therapy in later chapters.

2.3 Ecological Planetary Antifragility

The previous section offers what may be seen as an innovative ecological approach to cancer treatment by framing the tumor and its microenvironment as a complex, adaptive system similar, in some sense, to an ecosystem. In this context, cancer is

2.3 Ecological Planetary Antifragility

not merely a collection of rogue cells but an evolving entity that interacts dynamically with its surroundings, much like species within an ecosystem. This holistic perspective not only aims to maximize the tumor's response to treatment but also mirrors ecological management practices that prioritize resilience and adaptability over short-term gains, offering a promising path for developing more effective and sustainable cancer therapies.

Following the discussion about antifragility in medical treatment protocols, seen as an ecological problem, we now expand our focus to the broader end explicit problem of ecosystem antifragility, specifically on the planetary scale, examining how the principles of antifragility can inform our understanding of Earth's self-regulating systems and their capacity to adapt and thrive amid the challenges posed by climate change and biodiversity loss.

2.3.1 Introduction to Planetary Crisis and Antifragility

The current planetary crisis encompasses a range of pressing challenges, with climate change and biodiversity loss at the forefront. The Intergovernmental Panel on Climate Change (IPCC) warns that we are already experiencing the consequences of 1 °C of global warming, including extreme weather events and rising sea levels. Moreover, human activities have driven global temperatures 1 °C above pre-industrial levels, with projections indicating a likely 1.5 °C increase by 2030–2052 if current trends persist. Limiting warming to 1.5 °C is crucial, as even slight increases elevate the risk of irreversible changes, such as ecosystem loss.

Biodiversity loss compounds these challenges, with significant declines in species abundance and widespread extinctions, constituting what Dirzo has called Defaunation [29] that threatens both biodiversity and ecosystem functioning, exacerbating the planetary crisis. Additionally, Rockström and colleagues [30] identified nine planetary boundaries, including climate change and biodiversity loss, which delineate safe operating limits for human activities. Crossing these thresholds risks triggering irreversible tipping points in the Earth system, underscoring the urgency of collective action.

Figure 2.4 in the top-right sub-panel (based on [30] work) illustrates the precarious balance between safe margins and perilous overshoots in human activities, emphasizing the need for decisive global measures grounded in sound science. Addressing the planetary crisis demands immediate action to mitigate climate change, preserve biodiversity, and respect planetary boundaries. Only through a concerted effort can we navigate these challenges and secure a sustainable future for generations to come.

In this context of global change, ecology is the key field to understanding these problems and how we can cope with them. Nevertheless, unlike classical mechanics, which is described by Newton's Laws or Electromagnetic Theory described by Maxwell's equations, more than a century after it first appeared on the scene, Ecology today still seems to be too diverse and conflicted to be able to coalesce around any one coherent theory [15]. This lack of a core theoretical structure generates a lack of consensus in central concepts such as Ecosystem Health.

2.3.2 Theoretical Foundations

The quest for a unified theoretical framework in ecology has long been pursued, with efforts to establish fundamental principles akin to those found in classical physics. Ulanowicz [31] proposed the concept of increasing ascendency as a measure of system activity and organization within trophic exchanges. Drawing parallels to the extension of Newtonian laws by Schroedinger in formulating quantum physics, Ulanowicz suggests that increasing ascendency extends the principles of Newtonian mechanics into the realm of living systems, formulated as the ascendency principle: In the absence of major perturbations, ecosystems exhibit a propensity to increase in ascendency.

Regardless of the promising structure of ascendency, this assumption about the lack of major perturbations sets a non-trivial limitation for the full understanding of Ecosystem Health because part of it is related to ecosystem stability and the capacity of the ecosystems to respond to perturbations such as global impact due to anthropic activities.

In this perspective, Kleidon has proposed in [16] a re-conceptualization of Earth as a complex thermodynamic system, existing far from thermodynamic equilibrium by maximizing entropy production. The Maximum Entropy Production (MEP) concept applied to Earth system dynamics suggests that the planet engages in numerous energy-transforming processes, leading to a significant mass movement in the atmosphere, oceans, and on land, that enhance a self-organization in which eco-evolutionary processes take place. These local processes, however, may ultimately align with global biogeochemical processes outlined in [30].

In the same way, Michaelian [24, 25] has pointed out that ecosystems arise and evolve, as any other physical system, under the laws of thermodynamics. In particular, the relation between entropy production and ecosystem functioning up to the Earth system is well established and has been studied since 1972 in the pioneering work of Prigogine et al. [28] and then by Ulanowicz and Hannon [32], Aoki [33], Schneider and Kay [48], Schymanski et al. [49], Michaelian [24, 25, 50], Kleidon and Lorenz [34], Kleidon [35, 43–45], Kleidon et al. [46], and Panwar et al. [47].

This Earth's self-organizing nature has been outlined in the so-called Gaia Hypothesis, proposed by physicist James Lovelock and biologist Lynn Margulis in the 1970s [36, 41, 42].

The Gaian perspective suggests that the Earth functions as a system with dynamic interactions among both inorganic and organic components, which can self-regulate. Crucially, the organic living part of this system adapts to changing biogeochemical conditions within thermodynamic limits through the process of evolution by natural selection, while also influencing these conditions through its adaptations [28, 40].

2.3 Ecological Planetary Antifragility

Margulis and Lovelock suggested that Earth should have been experiencing continuous warming and increasing ocean acidity. However, the absence of such trends implies the presence of a planet-wide complex self-regulating system, where both planetary life and geological processes collaborate to stabilize climate and geology. Despite its significance, this concept remained untestable in the past due to its global scale.

In a recent work by Maull and co-workers [39], the authors describe a simplified representation of Earth's biosphere, to explore the concept of life-geosphere homeostasis in terms of the well-known Daisyworld model [51, 52] that illustrates how different species can adjust their populations in response to changes in the external environment, maintaining stable equilibrium. While Daisyworld exists only as a theoretical construct, the authors propose a real-world implementation using microbial consortia manipulated through genetic engineering. They suggest using pH as a control parameter and present theoretical and computational case studies involving two, three, and multiple species assemblies.

In a recent book [53], cognitive psychologist Arthur Reber, plant biologist Frantisek Baluska, and medical scientist William Miller challenge conventional notions of consciousness. They advocate for a paradigm shift that extends sentience not only to organisms but to the cellular level, positing that life and mind are inherently intertwined, a statement that could be seen as a manifestation of even a wider paradigm shift by seeing the world as evolving information [54].

From the cell, all the way through the development and subsequent evolution of the Earth's biodiversity have had profound biogeochemical ramifications. For instance, the emergence of vegetation cover altered the Earth's atmosphere composition, surface albedo, hydrological cycle, and nutrient availability. These changes created conducive conditions for further proliferation and diversification of life. This intricate and dynamic system persists despite significant external influences, such as the sequence of Croll-Milankovitch orbital cycles, which are thought to have triggered repeated ice ages and played a pivotal role in driving species diversification and range shifts, including the expansion of modern humans [37, 38]. In that way, it seems to be quite natural to construct a unifying framework that allows us to talk about how living complex systems respond to perturbation from the scale of cells to planets.

The Earth's self-organizing system, as depicted in the Gaia Hypothesis, can be viewed then as antifragile. This means that when faced with potentially catastrophic stressors, such as significant shifts in a planet's orbit, the system responds by continuously reorganizing and adapting, ultimately benefiting the system as a whole. Now the question is how can we measure planetary antifragility?

At this point, it is key to remember that antifragility is a contextual concept that is defined by the triplet system, perturbation, payoff function. The first element of the triplet has been discussed in the previous paragraphs, Gaia or the self-organizing Earth system. For the perturbation and the payoff function, a more detailed discussion is required.

Although in a very broad way we could consider anthropogenic global change as the perturbation, it might be necessary to highlight that human activities alone do not fully account for the current state of the Earth's systems. Rather, it is the hypercoupling of human activities with certain technologies that magnify their effects, resulting in what can be termed the Technocene [57, 62]. These technologies enable orders of magnitude more energy extraction and resource utilization than previously possible, leading to unprecedented environmental changes [60]. For instance, the energy flux in modern cities exceeds global primary productivity on land, underscoring the transformative impact of technology on Earth's systems.

In this context, the concept of the Anthropocene alone fails to capture the full extent of human-technological interactions and their implications for planetary dynamics. Instead, the Technocene framework offers a more comprehensive understanding of the current planetary crisis, acknowledging the role of technology as a central driver of environmental change. By incorporating a systems dynamics approach, we can better assess planetary antifragility in the face of technological perturbations, recognizing the complex interplay between human activities, technology, and the environment. Thus, understanding how living complex systems respond to perturbations at various scales, from cells to planets, requires considering the transformative power of technology in shaping Earth's systems in the Technocene era.

2.3.3 Measuring Planetary Antifragility

The concept of planetary antifragility, as we are presenting here based on our previous work [55], is rooted in very general thermodynamic arguments and offers a comprehensive framework for understanding ecosystem dynamics at various scales, from cells to planets [24, 25]. Ecosystems, like any other physical system, operate under the principles of thermodynamics, with entropy production serving as a reliable indicator of ecosystem health [28, 32–35, 43, 44, 46–49].

In our new Planetary Antifragility framework, inspired by the work of Michaelian [25], total entropy production per unit area of the ecosystem (J) is defined as the health indicator, given by the equation:

$$\text{Health} = J = \int_0^\infty 2\pi L_{rad}(\lambda) - 0.04 L_{in}(\lambda) \, d\lambda, \tag{2.13}$$

This equation encapsulates the entropy fluxes ($[Jm^{-2}K^{-1}]$) from both outgoing radiation ($L_{rad}(\lambda)$) and incoming solar radiation ($L_{in}(\lambda)$), where 2π accounts for isotropic emission and Lambertian reflection effects [5], and 0.04 represents the cosine of the incident radiation angle.

While measuring entropy production at a planetary scale requires a proxy that captures the most relevant information, satellite-based measurements of albedo anomalies offer a promising avenue [25, 32]. Albedo anomalies, representing deviations in surface reflectivity, reflect changes in energy fluxes and ecosystem dynamics at a global scale. By analyzing albedo data, we can approximate entropy production and assess planetary antifragility.

In the work on which we are basing this discussion (see Fig. 2.4 for a conceptual summary figure), we utilized published data on surface albedo anomalies in the Northern Hemisphere during July (GLASS albedo product) for the period 1981–2010 [22]. Following the approach of Ahmad et al. [61] for global mean temperature anomalies, we calculated the Fisher information of the albedo anomalies time series. The Fisher information quantifies the amount of information contained in a dataset and serves as a robust metric for assessing entropy production and ecosystem health.

In general, we consider albedo anomalies a valid proxy for entropy production, allowing us to quantify the payoff function for planetary antifragility.

Nevertheless, based on prior research into Ecosystem Antifragility [26], we have understood that assessing ecosystem health involves considering not only its state or integrity but also its dynamics. A healthy state occurs when ecosystems reach a level of complexity that enables self-organization, often characterized by criticality—a dynamic regime marked by scale invariance in Fourier space and equilibrium between informational emergence and self-organization [27].

Moreover, evidence starts to show that systems in criticality are also at maximum antifragility and exhibit maximum Fisher information [56], suggesting that Fisher information from core systemic variables, as in this case albedo, can serve as a more general proxy for antifragility.

2.3.4 Remarks

Considering the planet under the Gaian perspective of a self-organized system to maximum antifragility, it is clear that the standard concept of the "Safe Operating Space for Humanity" goes beyond merely defining state values for Planetary Boundaries. It involves acknowledging the significance of interactions among these boundaries and, notably, the dimension of perturbation response capacity for the Earth system.

This insight is related to recent work by Dudney and Suding [58], who emphasized that ecosystems rarely respond to environmental drivers in isolation. Incorporating interacting drivers may reveal more frequent threshold dynamics than previously recognized. Thus, our thermodynamic framework, utilizing global albedo as a proxy for planetary entropy production, can be seen as a systemic response that integrates all drivers and responses.

The use of Fisher Information as a measure of entropy production stability introduces the concept of homeostasis, reframed through time series analysis, as demonstrated by Fossion et al. [59] in a medical context. Healthy physiological processes, such as blood pressure regulation, involve coupling with other processes to absorb environmental variability. Similarly, ecosystem functions can be viewed as homeostatic processes maintained by fluctuations in species composition, suggesting that compositional shifts are more susceptible to threshold dynamics than ecosystem functions.

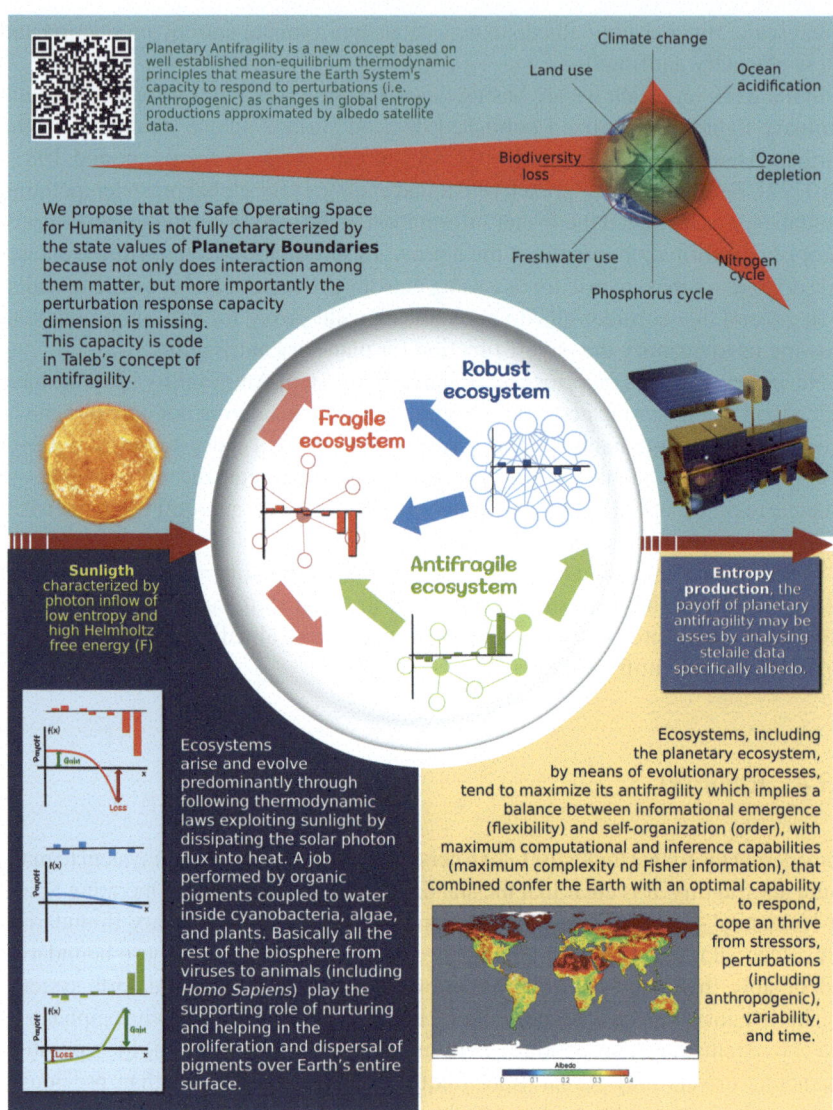

Fig. 2.4 Planetary antifragility is a new concept based on well-established non-equilibrium thermodynamic principles that measure the Earth system's capacity to respond to perturbations (i.e. anthropogenic) as changes in global Fisher information of entropy production (photon dissipation) approximated by albedo satellite data. Taken from [55] under Creative Commons Attribution 4.0 License

2.3 Ecological Planetary Antifragility

Interestingly, parallels can be drawn between Fossion's findings and Taleb's antifragility [67], prompting a reconceptualization of ecosystem homeostasis or resilience within Taleb's framework. Given that antifragility is quantitatively measured by the system's response to perturbation, we argue that planetary entropy production can be approximated by Earth's albedo.

By analyzing published data [22], we calculated Fisher Information for Northern Hemisphere albedo from 1988 to 2010. The observed oscillations in Fisher information values could suggest a cyclical decrease, potentially associated with human-induced perturbations like climate change and land use changes. This decrease indicates a loss of stability, overlapping with oscillations caused by changes in terrestrial albedo in response to teleconnected climate oscillations.

The overall decrease in Fisher Information implies that the planet is not only decreasing its albedo in response to human perturbations but also losing a crucial feature of its dynamics: its antifragility. This compounds the issue, as human perturbations such as climate change intensify while the planet loses its capacity to respond. Hence, efforts to address these challenges should not only focus on reducing or capturing CO_2 emissions but also on restoring Earth's antifragility, which necessitates restoring its ecosystems.

The current work faces several methodological limitations that warrant consideration. Firstly, while visible albedo is utilized as a proxy for global entropy production, it lacks standardized reference values akin to those in human health assessment. This absence necessitates determining reference values for each ecosystem type, requiring spatially explicit application of visible albedo rather than averaging mean values over large regions. Secondly, relying solely on visible albedo values overlooks their dynamics, analogous to assessing human health without considering dynamic physiological factors. To address this, the decision was made to utilize Fisher information, which captures the system's dynamics and its capacity to respond to perturbations. Thirdly, the measurement of ecosystem extent is influenced by the height of the remote sensor due to its relation with the solid angle of the detector, posing a challenge in accurately assessing the ecosystem's boundaries. Lastly, the instantaneous nature of albedo measurements underscores the need for integrating measurements over longer cycles to capture temporal variability adequately. Despite these considerations, the framework for Planetary Antifragility presented in this work remains underdeveloped, necessitating further exploration to determine if remote sensing measurements of albedo sufficiently capture entropy production or if additional signals are required, especially at more detailed scales.

Besides albedo, there is potential to integrate additional proxies for entropy production sources, offering avenues to address some of the limitations highlighted earlier. For instance, bioacoustic signals and ecosystem respiration present promising alternatives. Bioacoustic signals, emitted by various organisms within an ecosystem, encode valuable information about ecosystem metabolism. Particularly significant signals originate from members of the animal kingdom, providing insights that complement traditional measures like albedo. Moreover, ecosystem respiration, encompassing processes like soil respiration, offers a comprehensive proxy that reflects the intricate interactions across different environmental spheres. While projects like

Ameriflux collect ecosystem respiration data, the availability of planetary-scale data remains limited. Nonetheless, leveraging both remote sensing and in situ data can facilitate the downscaling of these concepts to the ecosystem level, enabling their integration into broader assessments of ecosystem health and integrity. (Reference: Ameriflux (https://ameriflux.lbl.gov/)).

Very interesting for us to realize that while introducing a new conceptual framework, the opportunity prompts us to reconsider the existing ecosystem paradigm, especially its definition, which is typically conceived as spatially explicit communities of living organisms interacting with their abiotic environment. However, as highlighted by Jax [23], managing ecosystems and advancing theoretical understanding necessitates a clear conceptualization, given the varied and sometimes conflicting definitions of ecosystems [17–21]. This ambiguity leads to challenging questions regarding the composition, dynamics, and stability of ecosystems, as well as their spatial extent and classification. Moreover, the definition's ability to address modified, degraded, or perturbed ecosystems and its applicability across different ecological contexts remains uncertain. Sagoff [18] emphasizes the need to refine ecosystem definitions to facilitate classification, model creation, causal identification, and problem-solving in socio-environmental contexts. Integrating the antifragility framework offers a promising avenue to address these challenges, potentially providing clarity on ecosystem boundaries and characteristics, thereby enhancing our understanding and management of ecosystems.

Under our novel framework, we define an ecosystem as an open thermodynamic system constituted by a community of living organisms in conjunction with the non-living components of their environment; that through its interactions and evolutionary processes, constrained by the external conditions; self-organized in a maximum solar photon flux dissipation, in which the system is at criticality, with maximum computational and inferential capabilities that allows it to respond and thrive under uncertainty, stressors, perturbations and ultimately time, in a well defined geographic context.

2.4 Neuronal Antifragility

The neuronal processing system is characterized by a high degree of complexity and subtlety, encompassing a vast array of dynamic processes. In the face of disturbances occurring over a range of timescales, from milliseconds to months or even years, neural networks must maintain stability. It may appear contradictory, but the only way neural networks can maintain stability is if they are excitable, capable of adapting their response (and structure) in response to external stimuli, and able to respond appropriately.

Like other biological systems, neural networks display a wide range of behaviors concerning modifications at the neuronal level, which regulate and enhance their functionality. They are capable of absorbing a diverse array of molecular and cellular parameter changes while maintaining their spiking functionality. However, the

2.4 Neuronal Antifragility

spectrum of behaviors is typically constructed with a strong reference to the basic state of stability. In this context, the term "stability" is used to describe the tendency of a dynamical system to return to its initial, steady-state equilibrium following the elimination of an input disturbance. This is characterized by the restoration of balanced relations between the system's components, including the post-spike refractory period and cell re-polarization.

We define robustness as the capacity of the system to withstand disturbances or variations in its input. Resilience can be defined as the ability of a system to regain its equilibrium once it experiences a variety of variations in parameters when these are tightly coupled. In this case, despite these modifications, the system reacts by modifying its internal states to preserve its general function. For instance, consider the excitability of individual neurons or neural networks that can withstand alterations in ionic channel expression, frequency of stimulation, temperature, salinity, and pH. Neurons are plastic and capable of adapting their behavior when faced with a new task, for example, an input pattern change concerning their frequency-current characteristic. This delineates the subsequent behavioral phenomenon, designated as "adaptation". This behavior is defined as the set of immediate adjustments in a cell or system (i.e. a neural network) triggered by a stimulus that persists.

2.4.1 Neural Correlates and Representations of Uncertainty

From the single neuron in the upstream section, uncertainty and volatility are explicitly encoded in several ways. The concept of uncertainty is considered an intrinsic feature of the environment, playing a pivotal role in the construction of internal models of decision-making and learning. In their study, [86] employed fMRI experiments to elucidate the encoding of uncertainty across diverse regions of the brain. The work defined pathways that modulate noradrenergic representations of uncertainty (i.e. risk, estimation uncertainty, unexpected uncertainty) in value-based decision-making using Bayesian tools. Building on this approach, volatility was conceptualized as a non-linear combination of the onset, duration and amplitude of external signal disturbances. This perspective is derived from the seminal study on imprecise neural computation as a source of adaptive behavior in volatile environments, as outlined in the seminal work of [89]. The study defined the statistical behavior in the presence of varying and fixed volatility models, leveraging three key elements: (1) high-order inferences about the environmental volatility, (2) neural computations that derive posterior beliefs, and (3) computational imprecision that scales with the magnitude of changes in internal representations.

In a broader context, it has been demonstrated that novelty and uncertainty act in concert to regulate exploration versus exploitation in the neural processing of risk [87] and ambiguity [88]. This is achieved either by employing a prediction error of uncertainty driving sensory learning, as observed in the work of [90], or by utilizing adaptive learning under expected and unexpected uncertainty, as evidenced by the findings of [91].

2.4.2 Robustness and Resilience in Neuronal Processing

Neuronal networks must be stable to maintain the learned relationships between the various sensory and motor streams they are modulated by and their internal states. From a dynamical systems perspective, such systems can only remain stable if they are excitable, able to adapt their behavior in reaction to external stimuli, and able to withstand those changes [64]. Conversely, neural networks are flexible, thereby exhibiting stability [135]. A network's capacity to accommodate minor variations in its parameters, operating variables, and state variables determines its overall stability [63]. In addition, a neuronal network is plastic and capable of adapting its behavior in response to new input configurations, tasks and noise patterns within its components and driving variables [65].

The concept of neuronal robustness and resilience can be observed across a range of scales, as illustrated by the example of feedback control systems [68]. Comprehensively and systematically, the authors present a behavioral spectrum, which encompasses a range of characteristics, from stability to adaptation, through to robustness and resilience. This represents the initial stage of our creative endeavour to expand the behavioral spectrum by incorporating a novel member, namely antifragility. This initiative is not merely theoretical; rather, it is based on previous research into the underlying mechanisms of robustness and resilience in neural systems. The current stability-resilience spectrum proposes that each behavior of single neurons and neural networks can be described as a seamless transition between multiple mechanisms that sustain function in the face of disruptions occurring on timelines spanning multiple orders of magnitude. This is due to the interleaving of distinct timescales, as suggested by the excellent framework of the comprehensive theory of adaptive variation [136].

The question thus arises as to how strategies and recovery mechanisms can be embedded in a mathematical framework for resilience dynamics under uncertainty while ensuring stable robustness. A noteworthy study of [121] proposed a definition of resilience as a form of controllability for entire random processes (regimes), whereby the state values must belong to an acceptable subset of the state set. To achieve this behavior, a combination of positive and negative feedback loops is required to sustain the propagation of the internal control signal under both functional and structural changes [124]. To achieve a comprehensive understanding of neuronal processing systems, it is essential to complement the dynamical analysis with formal measures of each behavior within the stability-resilience spectrum. In this regard, the study conducted by [125] illustrated that systems displaying feedback, nonlinearity, heterogeneity, and path dependencies must be represented in a unified mathematical framework. The study considered the Markov model framework provided above to establish formal definitions of several concepts in the dynamical systems behavior spectrum, including robust, reliable, sustainable, resilient, recoverable, stable, and static, as well as their counterparts: susceptible, vulnerable, and fragile.

2.4 Neuronal Antifragility

From a quantitative perspective, research has been conducted on the application of probabilistic techniques for the assessment of resilience in complex dynamical systems within feedback control loops. As emphasized in the study of [126], a feedback controller is responsible for system performance recovery through the application of different reconfiguration strategies and the strategic activation of necessary redundancy. Therefore, the impact of uncertainty and volatility on a system's operation is represented by disturbance factors. These observations are immediately applicable to the field of biological systems. In this regard, the study of [127] on resilience, reactivity, and variability offers a novel framework for understanding the spectrum of stable, robust, resilient, and adaptive behaviors. This framework is based on geometric eigenvector-based metrics, which capture time-scale separation and order reduction through eigenvector motion parameters.

The work of [128] employs a similar approach to that used in the geometrical framework of response shape in flow networks to introduce the concept of structural robustness. This is presented as the key to understanding the causal contribution of each system component to the network's robustness. This perspective is compatible with neuronal processing, as functional redundancy plays a fundamental role in the robustness and resilience of the system's response. This will be discussed in more detail later in the book in the context of its relationship to antifragility.

At last, the exhaustive study of resilience in dynamical systems by [69] presents a formal set of metrics and analytical techniques to elucidate the capacity of a dynamical system to accommodate alterations in state variables, driving variables, and parameters and to maintain its functionality. The framework was formalized using a concise set of metrics, including return time (reaching time, proportional to the reciprocal of the largest real part of the system's eigenvalues), reactivity (the maximum instantaneous rate at which an asymptotically stable linear system responds if initial conditions are away from the origin), and intrinsic stochasticity.

2.4.3 Robust Sensorimotor Control Under Uncertainty

It appears that the sensorimotor system has the inherent capability to enhance the reliability of its output in the presence of significant uncertainty. This is achieved by integrating sensory and motor information, each with distinct noise properties, in a manner that minimizes the overall estimate of uncertainty [84]. Such observations are even more accurately reflected in the framework of affordances discovery through perception and action [76], as also outlined in [75]. To be more precise, sensorimotor task performance is optimized by adapting the dynamics of the system under the prevailing physical and computational constraints [77].

In conclusion, the capacity to absorb changes in its parameters and input and recover from volatile disruptions remains within the realm of statistically optimal perception [78]. Even when formulated as feedback control loops, the computational models of sensorimotor integration continue to exploit the closed-loop dynamics to cope with noise in the input, disturbances and changes to the task structure. This is evidenced by the work of [79].

It appears that the stability-robustness-resilience-adaptiveness continuum in sensorimotor control also exhibits a hierarchical structure [80], which elucidates the interactions among the disparate time scales of sensory integration, motor plan generation, and disturbance compensation. This is particularly evident when considering the significant impact of coordinate transformation uncertainty [81]. A variety of explanations and models have been employed to elucidate the role of uncertainty in neural coding and computation underlying sensorimotor control [82]. Among these, Bayesian approaches to sensory integration [83] appear to be particularly prevalent.

However, none of the aforementioned approaches succeeds in capturing the consequences of fat tails [84], statistical moments and volatility [66], and the geometry of the system's response over time while learning under uncertainty [85].

2.4.4 Antifragility in Sensorimotor Processing

Experimental studies on mammalian brains have discovered that, on a local scale, these comprise similar structural features. Along those lines, the seminal work of American neurophysiologist Vernon Mountcastle proposed that the neuronal networks of the brain comprise large numbers of modules arranged in a columnar fashion. Moreover, his work suggested that these cortical columns expressed similar types of functionalities. It took several decades until neuroscientists gained closer insights into what functionalities these could constitute. Along those lines, South African neuroscientist Rodney Douglas and his colleagues showed evidence indicating that a core element of the cortical column implements soft winner-take-all functionality [138].

We anchor the explanations in a limited but representative set of neural sensorimotor control models to facilitate the conceptual work developed in this sub-chapter, based on the work in [116]. The initial studies that framed sensorimotor neuronal processing in control theory covered several classical aspects, including controllability and stabilization [108], observability and identification [107], and closed-loop feedback control [109].

In the present sub-chapter, we will analyze the characteristics of representative sensorimotor models through the lens of antifragility and its principal components. Our selection of models and the computational mechanisms is based on multiple recent computational and experimental studies that have emphasized the significant role of the "canonical" computational mechanisms (i.e., Homeostatic Activity Regulation—HAR, Winner Takes All—WTA, Hebbian Learning—HL) in neuronal processing behaviors. The study of [129] demonstrates that mitochondria play a pivotal role in the regulation of HAR. The release of synaptic vesicles and the intracellular calcium concentration were presented as examples of neuronal variables that are known to be regulated by mitochondria. The study developed a classification scheme for potential homeostatic machinery parts that stabilize firing rates by

2.4 Neuronal Antifragility

employing fundamental concepts from control theory, as depicted in Fig. 2.5. The study of [130] provides insights into the dynamical origin of WTA competition. The study employs a network of the hippocampus dentate gyrus to investigate the dynamic origin of WTA, which results in the sparse activation of the granule cell clusters. Under the findings of the dynamic systems analysis, the WTA dynamics can be attributed to a competition between the inhibitory cells' feedback and the firing activity within each cluster, schematically depicted in Fig. 2.6. A mathematical analysis of the effects of HL rules on the dynamics and structure of neural networks, as presented in the study by [131], offered valuable insights into the effects associated with a complex coupling between neuronal dynamics and synaptic graph structure. This approach provides a comprehensive understanding of the neural network evolution,

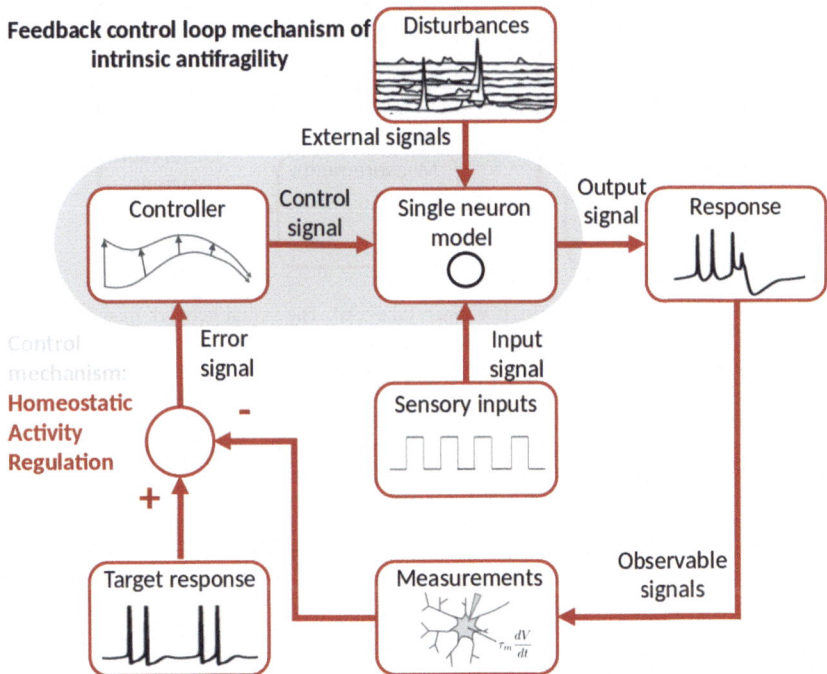

Fig. 2.5 Intrinsic antifragility through Homeostatic Activity Regulation. The single-neuron model of excitability follows a prescribed response (i.e., the target response) depending on the neuron type and function, for instance, bursting or tonic spiking. Here, the system to be controlled is the spike generation mechanism of the neuron model. At the same time, each neuron, based on its localization in the cortex, receives sensory input that will code in its spiking output. This always happens in the presence of disturbances (i.e., properties of the neuron, cross-talk with other neurons, and biochemical reactions in the neuron's environment). The neuron's response is a voltage that may be sensed, for instance, through changes in intracellular calcium levels, membrane voltage or pH. The fundamental component is the error signal, which represents the variation between the intended activity and the actual voltage response. The feedback controller then translates this error signal into a control signal, which controls the neuron's expression of its channel protein membrane

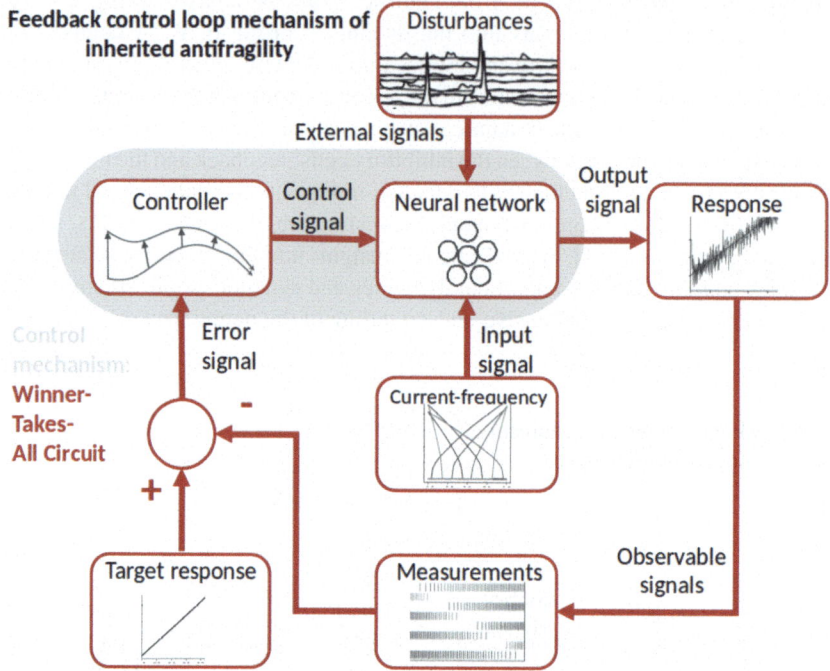

Fig. 2.6 Inherited antifragility through Winner Takes All. The neural network model encodes a specific input-output function with a prescribed shape (i.e., the target function) depending on the function of the network, for instance, sensory or motor. Here the system to be controlled is the neural network spiking pattern to generate the input-output function. This always happens in the presence of disturbances (i.e., properties of the composing neurons, cross-talk with other neurons). The network's response is a noisy version of the input-output function that may be sensed, for instance through changes in the output spiking frequency of the network's neurons. The fundamental component is the error signal, which represents the variation between the target function and the actual function spiking response. The feedback controller then translates this error signal into a control signal, which controls the neural network's update of synaptic connections among the neurons

encompassing both structural and dynamical perspectives, as captured in Fig. 2.7. From the perspective of Powell's perceptual control systems, and per the tenets of standard feedback control theory, the error signal, up to a certain degree, must be incorporated into the closed-loop behavior. More precisely, the ratio of the derivative of the error signal to the error signal itself indicates to the control system when an adjustment to the control signal is necessary but does not specify the precise manner or value of the adjustment. Furthermore, the rate of change of the error E, dE/dt, and its rate of change, d^2E/dt^2, inform the controller of the optimal timing and manner of control signal modification. These quantities can be conceptualized as degrees of freedom (DoF) provided by the external knowledge base. This is in line with the current developments in spiking control systems, where the event-based control

2.4 Neuronal Antifragility

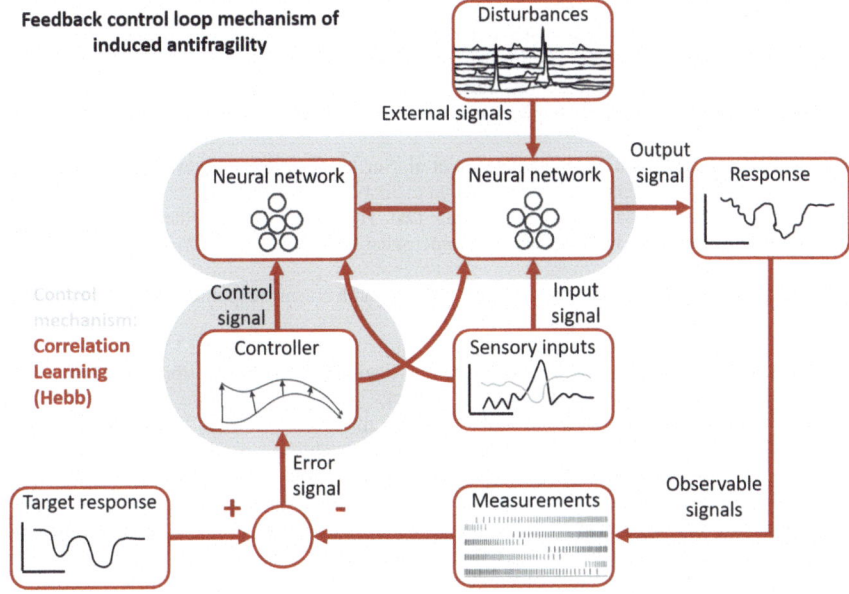

Fig. 2.7 Induced antifragility through Hebbian Learning. The neural network model encodes a specific cross-sensory or sensory-motor function with a prescribed shape (i.e., the target function) depending on the function of the interacting neural networks, for instance, coding for sensory or motor quantities. Here, the system to be controlled is the pair of neural networks spiking patterns to generate the joint cross-sensory or sensory-motor function. This always happens in the presence of disturbances (i.e., properties of the composing neurons, cross-talk within each neural network). Each neural network's response is a noisy version of the input-output function that may be sensed, for instance, through changes in the output spiking frequency of the network's neurons. This is then reflected in the accuracy of the cross-sensory or sensory-motor relation maintained among the two neural networks. The fundamental component is the error signal, which represents the variation between the target function and the actual function spiking responses of the two populations concerning the joint cross-sensory or sensory-motor function. The feedback controller then translates this error signal into a control signal, which controls both the neural networks' update of synaptic connections among the neurons

paradigm is unfolding over nested timescales [137]. In this context, positive feedback is responsible for enhancing or amplifying change, whereas negative feedback serves to dampen or buffer changes. The resulting mixed (positive/negative) controller acts as a monotone operator, which shapes the sensitivity of the closed-loop system and its excitability. This paradigm deviates from equilibrium designs and extends beyond robustness, aligning with the antifragile framework formulation.

References

1. Axenie, C., López-Corona, O., Makridis, M., Akbarzadeh, M., Saveriano, M., Stancu, A. & West, J. Antifragility as a complex system's response to perturbations, volatility, and time (2023).
2. Johan Ludwig William Valdemar Jensen et al. Sur les fonctions convexes et les inégalités entre les valeurs moyennes. *Acta mathematica*, 30:175–193, 1906.
3. MJ Piccart, Laura Biganzoli, and Angelo Di Leo. The impact of chemotherapy dose density and dose intensity on breast cancer outcome: what have we learned? *European Journal of Cancer*, 36:4–10, 2000.
4. Nassim Nicholas Taleb and Jeffrey West. Working with convex responses: Antifragility from finance to oncology. *Entropy*, 25(2):343, 2023.
5. Gates, D. M. (2012). *Biophysical ecology*. Springer Science & Business Media.
6. Robert S Kerbel and Barton A Kamen. The anti-angiogenic basis of metronomic chemotherapy. *Nature Reviews Cancer*, 4(6):423–436, 2004.
7. Jeffrey West, Bina Desai, Maximilian Strobl, Luke Pierik, Robert Vander Velde, Cole Armagost, Richard Miles, Mark Robertson-Tessi, Andriy Marusyk, and Alexander RA Anderson. Antifragile therapy. *BioRxiv*, pages 2020–10, 2020.
8. Dhara N Amin, Natalia Sergina, Deepika Ahuja, Martin McMahon, Jimmy A Blair, Donghui Wang, Byron Hann, Kevin M Koch, Kevan M Shokat, and Mark M Moasser. Resiliency and vulnerability in the her2-her3 tumorigenic driver. *Science translational medicine*, 2(16):16ra7–16ra7, 2010.
9. Jason I. Griffiths, Jinfeng Chen, Patrick A. Cosgrove, Anne O'Dea, Priyanka Sharma, Cynthia Ma, Meghna Trivedi, Kevin Kalinsky, Kari B. Wisinski, Ruth O'Regan, Issam Makhoul, Laura M. Spring, Aditya Bardia, Frederick R. Adler, Adam L. Cohen, Jeffrey T. Chang, Qamar J. Khan, and Andrea H. Bild. Serial single-cell genomics reveals convergent subclonal evolution of resistance as patients with early-stage breast cancer progress on endocrine plus cdk4/6 therapy. *Nature Cancer*, 2(6):658–671, 2021.
10. Christian Grommes, Geoffrey R Oxnard, Mark G Kris, Vincent A Miller, William Pao, Andrei I Holodny, Jennifer L Clarke, and Andrew B Lassman. "pulsatile" high-dose weekly erlotinib for cns metastases from egfr mutant non-small cell lung cancer. *Neuro-oncology*, 13(12):1364–1369, 2011.
11. M.A.R. Strobl, J. Gallaher, M. Robertson-Tessi, J. West, and A.R.A. Anderson. Treatment of evolving cancers will require dynamic decision support. *Annals of Oncology*, 34(10):867–884, 2023.
12. Renee Brady and Heiko Enderling. Mathematical models of cancer: When to predict novel therapies, and when not to. *Bulletin of Mathematical Biology*, 81(10):3722–3731, 2019.
13. Luke Pierik, Patricia McDonald, Alexander RA Anderson, and Jeffrey West. Second-order effects of chemotherapy pharmacodynamics and pharmacokinetics on tumor regression and cachexia. *Bulletin of Mathematical Biology*, 86(5):47, 2024.
14. Péter Bayer and Jeffrey West. Games and the treatment convexity of cancer. *Dynamic Games and Applications*, 13(4):1088–1105, 2023.
15. Ulanowicz, R. E. Some steps toward a central theory of ecosystem dynamics. Computational Biology and Chemistry, 27(6), 523–530 (2003).
16. Kleidon, Axel. "Nonequilibrium thermodynamics and maximum entropy production in the Earth system: applications and implications." Naturwissenschaften, vol. 96, no. 6, pp. 1–25, 2009. Springer.
17. Schaeffer, D. J., & Cox, D. K. (1992). Establishing ecosystem threshold criteria. In: Costanza, R., Norton, B. G., & Haskell, B. D. (Eds.), Ecosystem Health: New Goals for Environmental Management (pp. 157–169). Island Press, Washington, DC.
18. Sagoff, M. (2003). The plaza and the pendulum: Two concepts of ecological science. Biology and Philosophy, 18, 529–552. https://doi.org/10.1023/A:1025566804906
19. Jax, K. (2005). Function and "functioning" in ecology: what does it mean? Oikos, 111, 641–648. https://doi.org/10.1111/j.1600-0706.2005.13851.x

References

20. Jax, K. (2006). Ecological units: definitions and application. Quarterly Review of Biology, 81, 237–258. https://doi.org/10.1086/506237
21. Jax, K., Jones, C. G., and Pickett, S. T.: The self-identity of ecological units, *Oikos*, **82**, 253–264, 1998. https://doi.org/10.2307/3546965
22. He, T., Liang, S., Song, D.-X. (2014). Analysis of global land surface albedo climatology and spatial-temporal variation during 1981–2010 from multiple satellite products. Journal of Geophysical Research: Atmospheres, 119(17), 10281–10298. https://doi.org/10.1002/2014JD021667
23. Jax, K. (2007). Can we define ecosystems? On the confusion between definition and description of ecological concepts. Acta Biotheoretica, 55, 341–355. Springer.
24. Michaelian, Karo. "Thermodynamic stability of ecosystems." Journal of Theoretical Biology, vol. 237, no. 3, pp. 323–335, 2005. Elsevier.
25. Michaelian, Karo. "Photon Dissipation Rates as an Indicator of Ecosystem Health." Environmental Indicators, pp. 15–36, 2015. Springer.
26. Equihua, M., Aldama, M. E., Gershenson, C., López-Corona, O., Munguía, M., Pérez-Maqueo, O., Ramírez-Carrillo, E. (2020). Ecosystem antifragility: beyond integrity and resilience. PeerJ, 8, e8533. https://doi.org/10.7717/peerj.8533
27. Ramírez-Carrillo, E., López-Corona, O., Toledo-Roy, J. C., Lovett, J. C., de León-González, F., Osorio-Olvera, L., Equihua, J., Robredo, E., Frank, A., Dirzo, R., Pérez-Cirera, V. (2018). Assessing sustainability in North America's ecosystems using criticality and information theory. PLOS ONE, 13, e0200382. https://doi.org/10.1371/journal.pone.0200382
28. Prigogine, Ilya, Nicolis, Gregoire, and Babloyantz, Agnes. "Thermodynamics of evolution." Physics Today, vol. 25, no. 11, pp. 23–28, 1972. American Institute of Physics.
29. Dirzo, R., Young, H. S., Galetti, M., Ceballos, G., Isaac, N. J., and Collen, B. Defaunation in the Anthropocene. science, 345(6195), 401–406 (2014).
30. Rockström, Johan, Steffen, Will, Noone, Kevin, Persson, Åsa, Chapin III, F Stuart, Lambin, Eric, Lenton, Timothy M, Scheffer, Marten, Folke, Carl, Schellnhuber, Hans Joachim, et al. "Planetary boundaries: exploring the safe operating space for humanity". Ecology and Society, vol. 14, no. 2, 2009. JSTOR.
31. Ulanowicz, Robert E. "Life after Newton: an ecological metaphysic." BioSystems, vol. 50, no. 2, pp. 127–142, 1999. Elsevier.
32. Ulanowicz, R. E., Hannon, B. M. (1987). Life and the production of entropy. *Proceedings of the Royal Society of London. Series B, Biological Sciences*, *232*(1267), 181–192. Retrieved from http://www.jstor.org/stable/36217 (last access: July 22, 2022).
33. Aoki, I. (1989). Holological study of lakes from an entropy viewpoint Mendota. *Ecological Modelling*, *45*(1), 81–93. https://doi.org/10.1016/0304-3800(89)90085-9
34. Kleidon, A., Lorenz, R. D. (2005). *Non-equilibrium thermodynamics and the production of entropy: life, earth, and beyond*. Understanding Complex Systems.
35. Kleidon, A. (2009). Maximum entropy production and general trends in biospheric evolution. *Paleontological Journal*, *43*, 980–985. https://doi.org/10.1134/S0031030109080164
36. Lovelock, J. E. (1972). Gaia as seen through the atmosphere. *Atmospheric Environment*, *6*(8), 579–580.
37. Bennett, K. D. (1990). Milankovitch cycles and their effects on species in ecological and evolutionary time. *Paleobiology*, *16*, 11–21. https://doi.org/10.1017/S0094837300009684
38. Lovelock, J. E. (1989). Geophysiology, the science of Gaia. *Reviews of Geophysics*, *27*, 215–222. https://doi.org/10.1029/RG027i002p00215
39. Maull, V., Pla Mauri, J., Conde Pueyo, N., Solé, R. (2024). A synthetic microbial Daisyworld: planetary regulation in the test tube. *Journal of the Royal Society Interface*, *21*(211), 20230585. https://doi.org/10.1098/rsif.2023.0585
40. Lovelock, J. (2016). *Gaia: A new look at life on earth*. Oxford University Press, Oxford, UK.
41. Lovelock, J. E., Margulis, L. (1974). Atmospheric homeostasis by and for the biosphere: the Gaia hypothesis. *Tellus*, *26*(1-2), 2–10. https://doi.org/10.3402/tellusa.v26i1-2.9731
42. Margulis, L., Lovelock, J. E. (1974). Biological modulation of the Earth's atmosphere. *Icarus*, *21*(4), 471–489. https://doi.org/10.1016/0019-1035(74)90150-X

43. Kleidon, A. (2010a). Life, hierarchy, and the thermodynamic machinery of planet Earth. *Physics of Life Reviews*, *7*, 424–460. https://doi.org/10.1016/j.plrev.2010.10.002
44. Kleidon, A. (2010b). Non-equilibrium thermodynamics, maximum entropy production and Earth-system evolution. *Philosophical Transactions of the Royal Society A: Mathematical, Physical and Engineering Sciences*, *368*, 181–196. https://doi.org/10.1098/rsta.2009.0188
45. Kleidon, A. (2021). What limits photosynthesis? Identifying the thermodynamic constraints of the terrestrial biosphere within the Earth system. *Biochimica et Biophysica Acta (BBA) - Bioenergetics*, *1862*, 148303. https://doi.org/10.1016/j.bbabio.2020.148303
46. Kleidon, A., Malhi, Y., Cox, P. M. (2010). Maximum entropy production in environmental and ecological systems. *Philosophical Transactions of the Royal Society B: Biological Sciences*, *365*, 1297–1302. https://doi.org/10.1098/rstb.2010.0018
47. Panwar, A., Kleidon, A., Renner, M. (2020). What Cools Forests: Evaporation or Aerodynamic Conductance? En *AGU Fall Meeting Abstracts*, Vol. 2020, H192-05.
48. Schneider, E. D., Kay, J. J. (1994). Life as a manifestation of the second law of thermodynamics. *Mathematical and Computer Modelling*, *19*(6-8), 25–48. https://doi.org/10.1016/0895-7177(94)90188-0
49. Schymanski, S. J., Kleidon, A., Stieglitz, M., Narula, J. (2010). Maximum entropy production allows a simple representation of heterogeneity in semiarid ecosystems.
50. Michaelian, K. (2012). HESS Opinions "Biological catalysis of the hydrological cycle: life's thermodynamic function". *Hydrology and Earth System Sciences*, *16*(9), 2629–2645. https://doi.org/10.5194/hess-16-2629-2012 *Philosophical Transactions of the Royal Society B: Biological Sciences*, *365*(1545), 1449–1455. https://doi.org/10.1098/rstb.2009.0309
51. Watson AJ, Lovelock JE.Biological homeostasis of the global environment: the parable of Daisyworld. Tellus B 35, 284–289 (1983).
52. Lovelock JE, Watson AJ. The regulation of carbon dioxide and climate: gaia or geochemistry. Planet. Space Sci. 30, 795–802 (1982).
53. The Sentient Cell: The Cellular Foundations of Consciousness Arthur S. Reber, František Baluška, William B. Miller Jr. Oxford University Press, (2024).
54. Gershenson, C. The World as Evolving Information. In: Minai, A.A., Braha, D., Bar-Yam, Y. (eds) Unifying Themes in Complex Systems VII. Springer, Berlin, Heidelberg (2012).
55. López-Corona, O., Kolb, M., Ramírez-Carrillo, E., Lovett, J. (2022). ESD Ideas: planetary antifragility: a new dimension in the definition of the safe operating space for humanity. Earth System Dynamics, 13(3), 1145–1155.
56. López-Corona, O., & Padilla, P. (2019). Fisher information as a unifying concept for criticality and antifragility: A primer hypothesis. ResearchersOne. https://doi.org/10.13140/RG.2.2.28789.73444
57. Hamilton, C., Bonneuil, C., Gemenne, F. (2015). *The Anthropocene and the global environmental crisis: Rethinking modernity in a new epoch*. Taylor & Francis.
58. Dudney, J., & Suding, K. N. (2020). The elusive search for tipping points. Nature Ecology & Evolution, 4, 1449–1450. https://doi.org/10.1038/s41559-020-1273-8
59. Fossion, R., Rivera, A. L., & Estañol, B. (2018). A physicist's view of homeostasis: How time series of continuous monitoring reflect the function of physiological variables in regulatory mechanisms. Physiological Measurement, 39, 084007. https://doi.org/10.1088/1361-6579/aad8db
60. Burger, J. R., Weinberger, V. P., Marquet, P. A. (2017). Extra-metabolic energy use and the rise in human hyper-density. *Scientific Reports*, *7*(1), 43869. https://doi.org/10.1038/srep43869
61. Ahmad, N., Derrible, S., Eason, T., Cabezas, H. (2016). Using Fisher information to track stability in multivariate systems. Royal Society Open Science, 3(11), 160582. https://doi.org/10.1098/rsos.160582
62. Martins, H. (2018). *The Technocene*. Anthem Press.
63. Holling, C. Resilience and stability of ecological systems. *Annual Review Of Ecology And Systematics*. **4**, 1–23 (1973).
64. Cannon, W. Organization for physiological homeostasis. *Physiological Reviews*. **9**, 399–431 (1929).

References

65. Braun, E. The unforeseen challenge: from genotype-to-phenotype in cell populations. *Reports On Progress In Physics.* **78**, 036602 (2015).
66. Taleb, N. & Douady, R. Mathematical definition, mapping, and detection of (anti) fragility. *Quantitative Finance.* **13**, 1677–1689 (2013).
67. Taleb, N. Antifragile: Things that gain from disorder. (Random House Incorporated,2012).
68. Marom, S. & Marder, E. A biophysical perspective on the resilience of neuronal excitability across timescales. *Nature Reviews Neuroscience.* **24**, 640–652 (2023).
69. Krakovská, H., Kuehn, C. & Longo, I. Resilience of dynamical systems. *European Journal Of Applied Mathematics.* pp. 1–46 (2021).
70. Orbán, G. & Wolpert, D. Representations of uncertainty in sensorimotor control. *Current Opinion In Neurobiology.* **21**, 629–635 (2011).
71. Koblinger, Á., Fiser, J. & Lengyel, M. Representations of uncertainty: where art thou?. *Current Opinion In Behavioral Sciences.* **38** pp. 150–162 (2021).
72. Trommershäuser, J., Maloney, L. & Landy, M. Decision making, movement planning and statistical decision theory. *Trends In Cognitive Sciences.* **12**, 291–297 (2008).
73. Trommershäuser, J. Biases and optimality of sensory-motor and cognitive decisions. *Progress In Brain Research.* **174** pp. 267–278 (2009).
74. Körding, K. & Wolpert, D. Bayesian integration in sensorimotor learning. *Nature.* **427**, 244–247 (2004).
75. Beers, R., Baraduc, P. & Wolpert, D. Role of uncertainty in sensorimotor control. *Philosophical Transactions Of The Royal Society Of London. Series B: Biological Sciences.* **357**, 1137–1145 (2002).
76. Chavez-Garcia, R., Luce-Vayrac, P. & Chatila, R. Discovering affordances through perception and manipulation. *2016 IEEE/RSJ International Conference On Intelligent Robots And Systems (IROS).* pp. 3959–3964 (2016).
77. Ogawa, N., Sakaguchi, Y., Namiki, A. & Ishikawa, M. Adaptive acquisition of dynamics matching in sensory-motor fusion system. *Electronics And Communications In Japan (Part III: Fundamental Electronic Science).* **89**, 19–30 (2006).
78. Fiser, J., Berkes, P., Orbán, G. & Lengyel, M. Statistically optimal perception and learning: from behavior to neural representations. *Trends In Cognitive Sciences.* **14**, 119–130 (2010).
79. Ghahramani, Z., Wolptrt, D. & Jordan, M. Computational models of sensorimotor integration. *Advances In Psychology.* **119** pp. 117–147 (1997).
80. Nagata, S., Masumoto, D., Yamakawa, H. & Kimoto, T. Hierarchical Sensory-Motor Fusion Model with Neural Networks. *Journal Of The Robotics Society Of Japan.* **12**, 685–694 (1994).
81. Schlicht, E. & Schrater, P. Impact of coordinate transformation uncertainty on human sensorimotor control. *Journal Of Neurophysiology.* **97**, 4203–4214 (2007).
82. Knill, D. & Pouget, A. The Bayesian brain: the role of uncertainty in neural coding and computation. *TRENDS In Neurosciences.* **27**, 712–719 (2004).
83. Berniker, M. & Kording, K. Bayesian approaches to sensory integration for motor control. *Wiley Interdisciplinary Reviews: Cognitive Science.* **2**, 419–428 (2011).
84. Taleb, N. Statistical consequences of fat tails: Real world preasymptotics, epistemology, and applications. *ArXiv Preprint* ArXiv:2001.10488 (2020).
85. Topel, S., Ma, I., Sleutels, J., Steenbergen, H., Bruijn, E. & Duijvenvoorde, A. Expecting the unexpected: a review of learning under uncertainty across development. *Cognitive, Affective, & Behavioral Neuroscience.* pp. 1–21 (2023).
86. Payzan-LeNestour, E., Dunne, S., Bossaerts, P. & O'Doherty, J. The neural representation of unexpected uncertainty during value-based decision making. *Neuron.* **79**, 191–201 (2013).
87. Cockburn, J., Man, V., Cunningham, W. & O'Doherty, J. Novelty and uncertainty interact to regulate the balance between exploration and exploitation in the human brain. *BioRxiv.* pp. 2021-10 (2021).
88. Wu, S., Sun, S., Camilleri, J., Eickhoff, S. & Yu, R. Better the devil you know than the devil you don't: Neural processing of risk and ambiguity. *NeuroImage.* **236** pp. 118109 (2021).
89. Findling, C., Chopin, N. & Koechlin, E. Imprecise neural computations as a source of adaptive behaviour in volatile environments. *Nature Human Behaviour.* **5**, 99–112 (2021).

90. Iglesias, S., Kasper, L., Harrison, S., Manka, R., Mathys, C. & Stephan, K. Cholinergic and dopaminergic effects on prediction error and uncertainty responses during sensory associative learning. *NeuroImage*. **226** pp. 117590 (2021).
91. Soltani, A. & Izquierdo, A. Adaptive learning under expected and unexpected uncertainty. *Nature Reviews Neuroscience*. **20**, 635–644 (2019).
92. Grossman, C., Bari, B. & Cohen, J. Serotonin neurons modulate learning rate through uncertainty. *Current Biology*. **32**, 586–599 (2022).
93. Bach, D., Hulme, O., Penny, W. & Dolan, R. The known unknowns: neural representation of second-order uncertainty, and ambiguity. *Journal Of Neuroscience*. **31**, 4811–4820 (2011).
94. Van Bergen, R. & Jehee, J. Probabilistic representation in human visual cortex reflects uncertainty in serial decisions. *Journal Of Neuroscience*. **39**, 8164–8176 (2019).
95. Ma, W. & Jazayeri, M. Neural coding of uncertainty and probability. *Annual Review Of Neuroscience*. **37** pp. 205–220 (2014).
96. Bach, D. & Dolan, R. Knowing how much you don't know: a neural organization of uncertainty estimates. *Nature Reviews Neuroscience*. **13**, 572–586 (2012).
97. Muller, T., Mars, R., Behrens, T. & O'Reilly, J. Control of entropy in neural models of environmental state. *Elife*. **8** pp. e39404 (2019).
98. Friston, K., Shiner, T., FitzGerald, T., Galea, J., Adams, R., Brown, H., Dolan, R., Moran, R., Stephan, K. & Bestmann, S. Dopamine, affordance and active inference. *PLoS Computational Biology*. **8**, e1002327 (2012).
99. Feldman, H. & Friston, K. Attention, uncertainty, and free-energy. *Frontiers In Human Neuroscience*. **4** pp. 215 (2010).
100. Bland, A. & Schaefer, A. Different varieties of uncertainty in human decision-making. *Frontiers In Neuroscience*. **6** pp. 85 (2012).
101. Mushtaq, F., Bland, A. & Schaefer, A. Uncertainty and cognitive control. *Frontiers In Psychology*. **2** pp. 249 (2011).
102. Monosov, I. How outcome uncertainty mediates attention, learning, and decision-making. *Trends In Neurosciences*. **43**, 795–809 (2020).
103. Angela, J. & Dayan, P. Uncertainty, neuromodulation, and attention. *Neuron*. **46**, 681–692 (2005).
104. Schultz, W., Preuschoff, K., Camerer, C., Hsu, M., Fiorillo, C., Tobler, P. & Bossaerts, P. Explicit neural signals reflecting reward uncertainty. *Philosophical Transactions Of The Royal Society B: Biological Sciences*. **363**, 3801–3811 (2008).
105. Kosciessa, J., Lindenberger, U. & Garrett, D. Thalamocortical excitability modulation guides human perception under uncertainty. *Nature Communications*. **12**, 2430 (2021).
106. Weber, C. & Wermter, S. A self-organizing map of sigma–pi units. *Neurocomputing*. **70**, 2552–2560 (2007).
107. Levin, A. & Narendra, K. Control of nonlinear dynamical systems using neural networks: Controllability and stabilization. *IEEE Transactions On Neural Networks*. **4**, 192–206 (1993).
108. Levin, A. & Narendra, K. Control of nonlinear dynamical systems using neural networks. II. Observability, identification, and control. *IEEE Transactions On Neural Networks*. **7**, 30–42 (1996).
109. Narendra, K. Neural networks for control theory and practice. *Proceedings Of The IEEE*. **84**, 1385–1406 (1996).
110. Cook, M., Jug, F., Krautz, C. & Steger, A. Unsupervised learning of relations. *Artificial Neural Networks–ICANN 2010: 20th International Conference, Thessaloniki, Greece, September 15-18, 2010, Proceedings, Part I 20*. pp. 164–173 (2010).
111. Mandal, A. & Cichocki, A. Non-linear canonical correlation analysis using alpha-beta divergence. *Entropy*. **15**, 2788–2804 (2013).
112. Champion, K., Lusch, B., Kutz, J. & Brunton, S. Data-driven discovery of coordinates and governing equations. *Proceedings Of The National Academy Of Sciences*. **116**, 22445–22451 (2019).
113. Axenie, C. & Saveriano, M. Antifragile Control Systems: The Case of Mobile Robot Trajectory Tracking Under Uncertainty and Volatility. *IEEE Access*. **11** pp. 138188–138200 (2023).

References

114. Axenie, C. & Grossi, M. Antifragile Control Systems: The case of an oscillator-based network model of urban road traffic dynamics (2023).
115. Axenie, C., Kurz, D. & Saveriano, M. Antifragile Control Systems: The Case of an Anti-Symmetric Network Model of the Tumor-Immune-Drug Interactions. *Symmetry.* **14** (2022), https://www.mdpi.com/2073-8994/14/10/2034
116. Axenie, C. Antifragile control systems in neuronal processing: a sensorimotor perspective. *Biological Cybernetics.* **119**, 7 (2025).
117. Bruijn, H., Groessler, A. & Videira, N. Antifragility as a design criterion for modelling dynamic systems. *Systems Research And Behavioral Science.* **37**, 23–37 (2020).
118. Pineda, O., Kim, H., Gershenson, C. & Others A novel antifragility measure based on satisfaction and its application to random and biological Boolean networks. *Complexity.* **2019** (2019).
119. Pineda, O., Kim, H. & Gershenson, C. Antifragility of random Boolean networks (2018).
120. Kwon, Y. & Cho, K. Quantitative analysis of robustness and fragility in biological networks based on feedback dynamics. *Bioinformatics.* **24**, 987–994 (2008).
121. Lara, M. A mathematical framework for resilience: dynamics, uncertainties, strategies, and recovery regimes. *Environmental Modeling & Assessment.* **23**, 703–712 (2018).
122. Johnson, J. & Gheorghe, A. Antifragility analysis and measurement framework for systems of systems. *International Journal Of Disaster Risk Science.* **4** pp. 159–168 (2013).
123. Meyer, K. A dynamical systems framework for resilience in ecology. *ArXiv Preprint* ArXiv:1509.08175 (2015).
124. Hebbar, A., Moger, A., Hari, K. & Jolly, M. Interplay of positive and negative feedback loops governs robustness in multistable biological networks. *BioRxiv* (2022).
125. Bramson, A. Formal measures of dynamical properties: robustness and sustainability. *2010 AAAI Fall Symposium Series* (2010).
126. Balchanos, M. A probabilistic technique for the assessment of complex dynamic system resilience (2012).
127. Arnoldi, J., Loreau, M. & Haegeman, B. Resilience, reactivity and variability: A mathematical comparison of ecological stability measures. *Journal Of Theoretical Biology.* **389** pp. 47–59 (2016).
128. Ay, N. & Krakauer, D. Geometric robustness theory and biological networks. *Theory In Biosciences.* **125** pp. 93–121 (2007).
129. Ruggiero, A., Katsenelson, M. & Slutsky, I. Mitochondria: new players in homeostatic regulation of firing rate set points. *Trends In Neurosciences.* **44**, 605–618 (2021).
130. Kim, S. & Lim, W. Dynamical origin for winner-take-all competition in a biological network of the hippocampal dentate gyrus. *Physical Review E.* **105**, 014418 (2022).
131. Siri, B., Berry, H., Cessac, B., Delord, B. & Quoy, M. A mathematical analysis of the effects of Hebbian learning rules on the dynamics and structure of discrete-time random recurrent neural networks. *Neural Computation.* **20**, 2937–2966 (2008).
132. Pedersen, J., Abreu, S., Jobst, M., Lenz, G., Fra, V., Bauer, F., Muir, D., Zhou, P., Vogginger, B., Heckel, K. & Others Neuromorphic Intermediate Representation: A Unified Instruction Set for Interoperable Brain-Inspired Computing. *ArXiv Preprint* ArXiv:2311.14641 (2023).
133. Firouzi, M., Glasauer, S. & Conradt, J. Flexible Cue Integration by Line Attraction Dynamics and Divisive Normalization. *Artificial Neural Networks And Machine Learning–ICANN 2014: 24th International Conference On Artificial Neural Networks, Hamburg, Germany, September 15-19, 2014. Proceedings 24.* pp. 691–698 (2014).
134. Axenie, C., Richter, C. & Conradt, J. A self-synthesis approach to perceptual learning for multisensory fusion in robotics. *Sensors.* **16**, 1751 (2016).
135. Musslick, S., Bizyaeva, A., Agaron, S., Leonard, N. & Cohen, J. Stability-flexibility dilemma in cognitive control: A dynamical system perspective. *Proceedings Of The 41st Annual Meeting Of The Cognitive Science Society* (2019).
136. Meyers, L. & Bull, J. Fighting change with change: adaptive variation in an uncertain world. *Trends In Ecology & Evolution.* **17**, 551–557 (2002).
137. Sepulchre, R. Spiking control systems. *Proceedings Of The IEEE.* **110**, 577–589 (2022).

138. Douglas, R., Martin, K. & Whitteridge, D. A canonical microcircuit for neocortex. *Neural Computation*. **1**, 480–488 (1989).
139. Wikimedia Commons. (2015). *Planetary boundaries 2015* [Diagram]. Retrieved from https://commons.wikimedia.org/wiki/File:Planetary_Boundaries_2015.svg

Chapter 3
Evolutionary Antifragility

Abstract This chapter introduces evolutionary antifragility as the time-scale interaction characteristics of a natural dynamic system. It describes the benefit derived from input distribution unevenness, based on the emergent system dynamics and its uncertain and volatile interactions with the operating environment described by unknown disturbances. We consider methods for the detection, analysis, and modelling of cancer, environmental, microbiota, and social systems antifragility.

3.1 Defining Evolutionary Antifragility

The previous chapter has illustrated the connection between the convexity of the payoff function, $f(x)$, and the outcome benefit to input variation. Here, we extend this idea to illustrate the connection between convexity and the statistical properties of the distribution of $f(x)$. There are many biological systems for which it is difficult to measure the system's response function. Alternatively, the system's payoff function may indeed be well-characterized, but external signals or noise introduce additional, unpredictable nonlinearities. We will illustrate several examples of observed antifragile behavior in the outcome distributions despite an unknown or unmeasurable response function.

3.2 Probability Convolution for Convex and Concave Functions

We begin with a simple example function and use probability convolution methods to derive the exact expression of this outcome distribution of $f(x)$, given some input probability distribution of x. These probability distribution functions (p.d.f.)

will have associated properties depending on if the underlying function is convex, concave, or linear. Consider the following function:

$$f(x) = x^c \tag{3.1}$$

where c is a constant. As seen in Fig. 3.1a, the shape of this function can be convex ($c > 1$; blue), concave ($c < 1$; red), or linear ($c = 1$; black). Let $p(x)$ be the probability density function describing the input distribution of x. For example, Fig. 3.1b shows a normal distribution with corresponding μ, σ: $p(x) = N(\mu, \sigma)$:

$$p(x) = \frac{1}{\sigma\sqrt{2\pi}} e^{-\frac{1}{2}\left(\frac{x-\mu}{\sigma}\right)^2}. \tag{3.2}$$

The probability density function of the outcome, $f(x)$, can be determined by convolution. Let X be a random variable (input) and let $y(X) = f(X)$, then the outcome distribution of $f(x)$ is given by:

$$P(y(a) \leq Y < y(b)) = \int_a^b p(x)dx \tag{3.3}$$

$$= \int_{y(a)}^{y(b)} p(x(y)) \left|\frac{dx}{dy}\right| dy \tag{3.4}$$

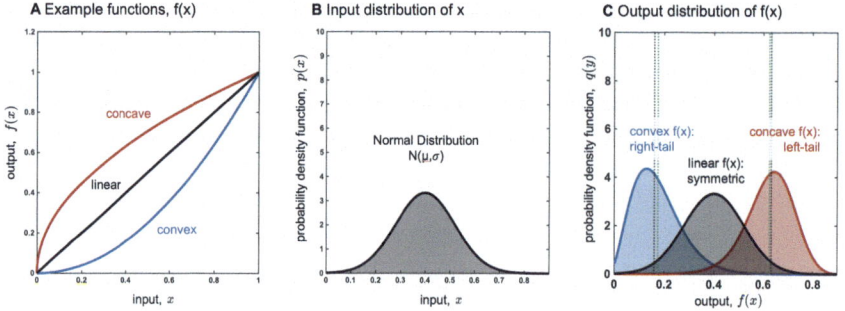

Fig. 3.1 a Three example functions are shown. Blue: convex function where $f(x) = x^2$. Red: concave function $f(x) = x^{\frac{1}{2}}$. Black: linear function where $f(x) = x$. **b** Consider a continuous random variable, **X**, which has an associated probability density function that is normally distributed with mean $\mu = 0.4$ and standard deviation $\sigma = 0.12$. **b, c** We plot the probability density function representing the distribution of outcomes, $f(x)$ for the corresponding convex (blue), concave (red), and linear (black) in A. For convex functions (**b**), the right tail drives the mean of the outcome distribution up so that $\mathbb{E}(f(x)) > f(\mathbb{E}(x))$. For concave functions, the left tail drives the mean down, so that $\mathbb{E}(f(x)) < f(\mathbb{E}(x))$. For linear functions, the outcome distribution is symmetric (no tail)

3.3 Evolutionary Antifragility in Medicine

where the argument inside the integral is the p.d.f. of $f(x)$, which we denote as $q(y)$:

$$q(y) = p(x(y)) \left| \frac{dx}{dy} \right|. \tag{3.5}$$

For the example function $f(x)$ given above, both terms of the integrand can be found analytically:

$$x(y) = y^{\frac{1}{c}}, \tag{3.6}$$

and

$$\left| \frac{dx}{dy} \right| = \frac{1}{c} y^{\frac{1-c}{c}}, \tag{3.7}$$

which gives:

$$q(y) = \frac{y^{\frac{1-c}{c}}}{\sigma c \sqrt{2\pi}} e^{-\frac{1}{2}\left(\frac{y^{\frac{1}{c}}-\mu}{\sigma}\right)^2}. \tag{3.8}$$

The key parameter is c, which determines the tailedness of the outcome distribution, as shown in Fig. 3.1c. Convex functions ($c > 1$) are associated with right tails, which cause an increase in the mean of the distribution, such that $\mathbb{E}(f(x)) > f(\mathbb{E}(x))$. Concave functions ($c < 1$) are associated with a left-tail, leading to the opposite conclusion: $\mathbb{E}(f(x)) < f(\mathbb{E}(x))$. The implications for systems where the system response function $f(x)$ is unknown are important. Because of the nature of probability distributions, everything fragile (left-tailed) must be concave, while everything antifragile (right-tailed) must be convex [1]. Thus, it's possible to determine the benefit (or harm) from input variation through knowledge of the tailedness of the outcome distribution, without knowledge of the underlying functional response, $f(x)$. In the following sections, we illustrate an example of this approach in medicine.

3.3 Evolutionary Antifragility in Medicine

3.3.1 *Inferring (Anti)-Fragility from Kaplan-Meier Curves*

Kaplan-Meier (KM) curves are ubiquitous in clinical trials to determine the efficacy of novel drugs or treatment protocols. KM curves show the fraction of patients who have not yet experienced disease progression, as a function of time [2]. In this example, we model a single patient's time to progression (TTP) and illustrate the differences in KM curves across an entire patient cohort when the underlying functional relationship between dose sensitivity and TTP is either convex, concave, or linear (see Fig. 3.2).

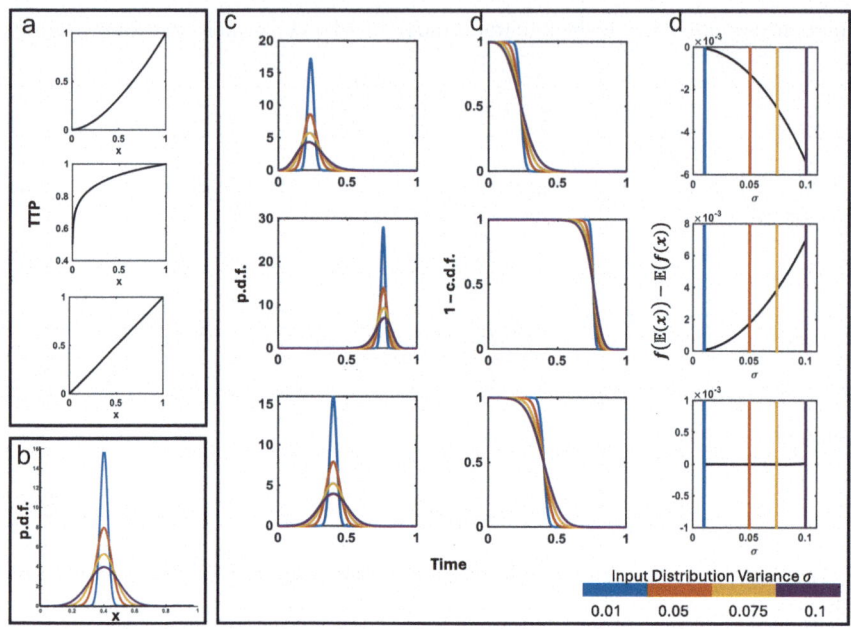

Fig. 3.2 a Input response function, for an input function $f(x) = x^c$, the convexity of the result can be determined via manipulation of c. The result is one of three potential outcomes: convex, concave, or linear. **b** Dose distribution p.d.f., Given the previous input function, we can state that the mean dose administered is $\mathbb{E}(x) = 0.4$. Simply by changing the observed standard deviation (σ) of the p.d.f., we can see a variety of potential for the dose received. **c** Outcome distribution p.d.f. and resulting Kaplan Meier (**d**), this can be expanded to observations within the tailedness of the outcome distribution p.d.f. When input functions are convex, the resulting outcome distribution will be right-tailed. Conversely, the opposite will be seen when input functions are concave. **e** Comparison of Jensen's gap. Within nonlinear functions, due to the convexity/concavity of the function: $f(\mathbb{E}(x)) \geq \mathbb{E}(f(x))$ or $f(\mathbb{E}(x)) \leq \mathbb{E}(f(x))$ respectively, will be true due to Jensen's inequality. In linear functions, $\mathbb{E}(f(x))$ and $f(\mathbb{E}(x))$ are identical, and thus, Jensen's gap is zero for all values of σ

Let X be a random variable (dose sensitivity, x) and let the $y(X) = f(X)$ represent the time to progression as a function of dose sensitivity:

$$f(x) = x^c. \tag{3.9}$$

In the previous section, we have performed the analytical solution of the convolution of the system response function, $f(x)$, and the input p.d.f., $p(x)$ (see Eq. (3.2)) and its corresponding c.d.f (see eqn. (3.8)). Consider the three types of functions in Fig. 3.2a (convex, concave, linear), with associated input variance, $p(x)$ (Fig. 3.2b). Here, the variance in dose, x, represents the inter-patient differences in drug delivery, tumor sensitivity, and other sources of patient-to-patient heterogeneity in drug response. We show the resulting p.d.f in Fig. 3.2c. By integrating the p.d.f., we can plot the KM curve (equivalent to 1− c.d.f. with no censoring) shown in Fig. 3.2d. This approach is similar to previous frameworks that primarily utilize numerical methods to convolve inter- and inter-patient variation in drug sensitivity to fit KM curves [3, 4]. The advantage of the approach shown here is that the analytical relationship between the input distribution, $p(x)$ and output distribution, $q(y)$, is known and does not require numerical approximation.

While KM curves are considered the gold standard of medical trial reporting, information can often visually obscure the tailedness of the underlying distribution. In Fig. 3.2d, increasing the value of σ does not shift the inflection point (the time at which 50% of patients have progressed), but there are differences before and after this inflection. These are better illustrated in the corresponding p.d.f (Fig. 3.2c), where the resulting tailedness is noticeably different. As expected, convex functions are right-tailed, while concave functions are left-tailed, and linear functions are perfectly symmetric about the mean.

In a treatment context, this can be explained through the importance of extreme dose sensitivity (both high and low) and its effect on outcome. For a given population's drug sensitivity (mean and variance), if the therapeutic benefit has decreasing returns as dose increases as in a concave response, extreme doses would contribute overall less to the mean value of the therapeutic outcome. Conversely, convex dose response outlier patients will amplify the population's mean responsiveness, especially when input variance is larger. The difference in the mean values (e.g. the antifragility) can be quantified as follows:

$$f(\mathbb{E}(x)) - \mathbb{E}(f(x)) = \mu^c - \int_{-\infty}^{\infty} yq(y)dy \tag{3.10}$$

The differences are shown in Fig. 3.2e, confirming that this difference is positive (antifragile) for convex functions, negative (fragile) for concave functions and zero for linear functions. Therefore, by understanding the underlying distribution function and its variability, the tradeoff between efficacy and safety, as well as risk, can be better assessed. This would then allow for a better understanding of how variability impacts the desired clinical outcome. It can be used to inform dosing strategies for personalized medicine applications. When the underlying input distribution is known (or can be estimated), the resulting p.d.f. of outcomes can be obtained from just a KM curve via backward convolution.

3.3.2 Current Applications in Medicine

These concepts can directly tie to the clinical practice of adaptive therapy, in which the prescribed dosing of treatment is continuously adjusted based upon tumor evolution and disease progression [5]. Adaptive therapy is not used as an extinction therapeutic but more commonly as a way for disease management/control while maintaining a high degree of quality of life [6, 7]. Dose modulations are designed to promote cell-cell competition among sensitive and resistant cell populations [5, 8]. The key difference between adaptive therapy and standard-of-care approaches is the increased variance in dose delivered [9]. The benefits arising from input perturbations illustrate how adaptive therapy's underlying philosophy is related to antifragility. By allowing for perturbations, patient response can be seen to be increasingly positive while maintaining other clinically important factors (e.g. limiting resistance emergence).

Many conditions outside of cancer can likewise be improved through perturbations to the environment. One such example is the application of radiotherapy in patients with Osteoarthritis (OA). Characterized by a decrease in mobility and increasing pain and stiffness of joints, current treatment options for OA range from lifestyle modification to total joint arthroplasty. Radiotherapy provides an alternative, minimally invasive option with proven success where low-dose application was used (a dose of 0.5Gy per fraction for 6 fractions given every other day or twice weekly) [10–12]. These small environmental perturbations allow for multiple mechanisms of anti-inflammatory effects, such as an increase in anti-inflammatory cytokines (e.g. IL10, TGF-β1), decreased production of reactive oxygen species, and increased polarization of Macrophages to the M2-phenotype [13].

The benefit to the patient lies not only in the therapies' mechanism of action but also its schedule. Previous work applied antifragile theory to measure second-order effects on resistance, collateral sensitivity, and combination treatments [14]. In the context of resistance, there is an expanded range of dose values classified as antifragile after the evolution of resistance has occurred [14]. This would indicate that treatment schedules with increased perturbations are more beneficial. This effect is exaggerated when accounting for pharmacokinetics and drug delivery [15]. For collateral sensitivity, it is possible to maintain secondary vulnerabilities to a subsequent therapy line. This is supported in part by the shifting of cell lines from fragile to antifragile responses during treatment.

3.4 Threshold Effects Lead to Antifragility

We now illustrate how threshold effects lead to antifragility. A step function (Fig. 3.3a) has no response below a certain threshold value, h. A step function is antifragile to an increase in variance because it is convex. Consider the effect of increasing the input distribution variance in Fig. 3.3b, where low variance leads to zero probability (Fig. 3.3b, top), but high variance extends the right tail to exceed the threshold value.

This scenario is widely applicable in natural systems. For example, BT crops that have been genetically modified to produce a constant level of pesticide still perform worse when compared to occasional manual interventions by farmers [16]. This is because the pesticide self-production by these crops is lower than the threshold required to affect pests. Occasion intervention dramatically increases the variance (e.g. weekly or monthly), but each intervention exceeds the required threshold for

3.5 We Are Not Trees but Forests

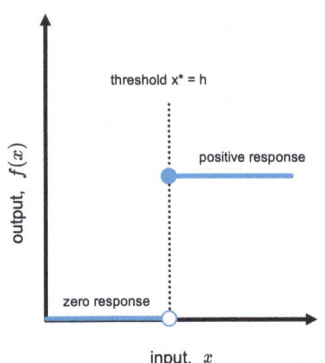
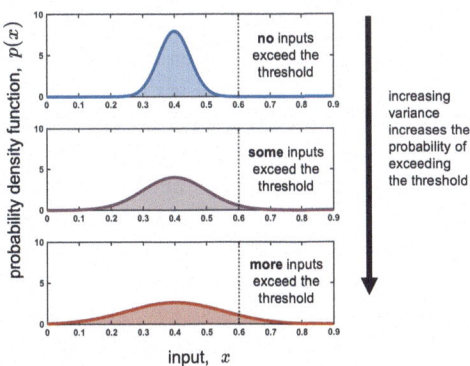

Fig. 3.3 Relationship between input distribution variance and threshold effects. Assume an input distribution (e.g. Normal distribution with associated mean μ and variance σ and some threshold value, $x^* = h$ such that $h > \mu$. As variance increases, the likelihood of observing events that exceed the threshold also increases

response. Other examples in nature include stochastic resonance, where stochastic noise increases the signal's response to rising above the threshold of detection [76].

The role of variance is also known to be important in evolutionary medicine. Recent approaches in antibiotics [17, 18] and cancer therapy [5, 6, 19, 20] have drawn inspiration from agricultural practices of periodic pesticide administration to avoid resistance. In this case, increasing the variance of dose delivered through pulsatile or periodic administration reduces the cumulative dose *below* a desired dose threshold, above which resistance occurs [9]. A high dose targets the treatment-sensitive clones within a tumor, leading to the competitive release of treatment-resistant clones and rapid expansion of resistance [8, 21]. Observing the concavity of the dose-response curve in ovarian cancer has shown promise in designing treatment scheduling with reduced variance while at the same time lowering the cumulative dose [22].

3.5 We Are Not Trees but Forests

Let us remember that when talking about Antifragility, we need to specify the triplet {system, payoff function, perturbation}.

In that sense, Alejandro Frank uses the phrase "We are not trees but forests" which encapsulates the idea that humans, like forests, are not singular entities, individuals or trees, but rather complex ecosystems comprised of symbiotic relationships with myriad microorganisms.

3.5.1 Evolutionary Implications of the Holobiont Concept

As explained by Huitzil and co-workers [23], this concept challenges the traditional view of organisms in isolation and emphasizes the importance of considering the collective entity of host and microbiota, known as the holobiont [45]. Within this framework, the microbiome, encompassing the genetic material of all microorganisms associated with a host organism, emerges as a critical component shaping the host's phenotype, physiology, and adaptive potential [56, 57]. Just as forests are composed of diverse flora and fauna interacting in complex ways, humans harbour a vast array of microorganisms that profoundly influence various aspects of their biology.

By acknowledging the holobiont as the fundamental unit of evolutionary analysis, we can gain insights into unresolved questions in evolutionary biology, such as rapid evolution and the missing heritability problem [32–34]. Recent evidence suggests that the microbiome contributes significantly to host adaptation and inheritance, challenging conventional genetic frameworks [24, 35, 36]. Simulation-based studies have demonstrated that host-microbiome interactions can enhance host adaptation and generate phenotypic variability beyond what can be explained by host genetics alone [25]. These findings underscore the importance of considering the microbiome as a source of variation subject to natural selection, thus expanding our understanding of inheritance mechanisms.

Furthermore, the concept of the holobiont emphasizes the interdependence of host-microbiome interactions, highlighting the need for a more inclusive interpretation of inheritance that incorporates non-genetic factors [36, 46, 55]. This holistic perspective offers a paradigm shift from the reductionist view of genetics to a more integrative framework that encompasses the microbiome's role in evolutionary processes [31, 47]. Ultimately, recognizing humans as holobionts underscores the complexity and interconnectedness of biological systems, providing a foundation for addressing key challenges in evolutionary biology and advancing our understanding of organismal evolution.

It is clear then that the gut microbiota function as a rapid response subcontrol system within the holobiont and working alongside the host genome, a slow response subcontrol system, enhances the holobiont's ability to achieve eco-evolutionary criticality and maximum antifragility control system as in our general applied antifragility framework.

Rapid evolution, characterized by swift adaptation to novel environments in fewer generations than predicted by traditional evolutionary models, has been attributed to various mechanisms, including phenotypic plasticity, epigenetics, and speciation facilitated by microbial interactions [26–28]. The microbiome's capacity to introduce new genetic material, modify gene expression, and induce reproductive barriers between populations contributes to phenotypic variation and rapid adaptation in holobionts [28–30]. Additionally, alterations in the microbiome composition serve as a significant driver of rapid adaptation, influencing allele frequencies and genome-wide differentiation in host populations [28]. Through direct and indirect pathways, the microbiome plays a crucial role in guiding host evolution by responding rapidly to environmental changes and shaping the fitness landscape of natural populations [37].

The rapid evolutionary shifts observed in the infant gut microbiome following birth underscore the microbiome's proactive role in host adaptation, potentially affecting lineage persistence and gut microbiome development [48]. Moreover, human microbiomes have undergone expedited changes from ancestral states, indicating their involvement in the rapid evolution of humans, particularly in response to dietary shifts and environmental factors [49]. Correlational evidence from diverse ecosystems, including corals, fish, and bacteria, highlights the active contribution of microbial communities to host adaptation, emphasizing the need for further investigation into the microbiome's role in rapid evolution [50–52]. While correlational studies provide valuable insights, definitive relationships between microbial interactions and host adaptation require integrated frameworks that combine mathematical modeling with the holobiont concept [53].

Our proposed integrative approach combines mathematical models with the holobiont concept to elucidate the mechanisms underlying microbial interactions and their contribution to host adaptation. By incorporating insights from previous research and exploring the evolutionary consequences of the holobiont concept, we aim to develop a unified model that comprehensively explains the microbiome's role in driving rapid evolution within holobionts. Through collaborative efforts and interdisciplinary approaches, we can achieve a deeper understanding of the microbiome's impact on host evolution, ultimately advancing our knowledge of eco-evolutionary dynamics and enhancing the antifragility of holobionts [54].

3.5.2 The Microbiota-Gut-Brain Axis as a Model for Antifragility

An excellent model for studying the holobiontic antifragility is the microbiota-gut-brain axis, which is composed of a wide variety of microorganisms and plays a fundamental role in human health and homeostasis [63]. In addition to contributing to nutrition, metabolism, and host protection, the intestinal microbiota also participates in the bidirectional communication between the gastrointestinal tract and the central nervous system through the gut-brain axis [63]. This interaction has a significant impact on a variety of health and disease processes, including neurological disorders, highlighting the importance of understanding the dynamics of this ecosystem [31].

Studying the microbiota-gut-brain axis from an ecology and complexity perspective allows for a better understanding of how interactions between the intestinal microbiota and the human brain influence health and cognitive functioning [67]. For example, stress has been shown to affect the composition and activity of the intestinal microbiota, which can, in turn, influence the response to stress, anxious behaviors, and activation of the hypothalamic-pituitary-adrenal stress axis [69]. This complex gut-brain communication network modulates both gastrointestinal functions and aspects of mood and cognition, underscoring the need to understand the interactions between these systems at different levels of scale [57].

As we discuss in chapter two, one can characterise the health of the human microbiota ecosystem by its integrity, which emerges from self-organization and emergent processes operating through locally existing biota [82]. The criticality of this ecosystem and its ability to respond and adapt to perturbations or even improve in the face of stress and disturbances is the axis antifragility. Recent studies have shown that certain disturbances, such as the presence of parasites, can reduce the criticality of the intestinal microbiota, affecting its responsiveness to environmental stressors [84].

In terms of the antifragility triplet of {system, payoff function, perturbation}, once we defined the system as the microbiota-gut-brain axis, then we have to identify an adequate payoff function, which is a methodological change since we are considering two very different components: the gut microbiota ecosystem and the brain functioning, so how could we asses both subsystems antifragility with a single metric?

Achieving maximum antifragility in living systems necessarily implies the most efficient transmission of multiscale information possible. Network Theory Methods (NTM) have emerged as valuable tools in understanding the complexity of biological systems, particularly in neurobiological studies [63, 65–67]. However, traditional network metrics like node centrality indices may lack scale invariance, posing limitations in measuring complex systems. To address this, Saba and colleagues [62] advocate for the use of the Minimum Spanning Tree (MST), which considers both topological properties and functional connectivity information. MST, a well-studied optimization problem in computer science, calculates a tree connecting all vertices of a network with the minimum total weight among all possible spanning trees. This approach enables a multidisciplinary analysis of biological components, such as the brain and gut microbiota (GM), as interconnected complex systems, providing a straightforward and computable method to assess information transmission efficiency.

3.5.3 Impact of Diet and Lifestyle on Holobiont Antifragility

Following these ideas [44], we employ this complex system approach to investigate how protein and lipid consumption in children may influence the connectivity of brain cortex activity (BCA) and GM. We focus on an indigenous Mexican community, the Me'phaa, residing in a region with distinct lifestyle characteristics compared to urbanized areas [58, 64, 75]. Subsistence farming dominates their diet, with limited access to animal-based products, resulting in significant interindividual variation in nutrient intake [68]. This community presents a unique model to study the impact of nutritional diversity on GM and BCA networks, as it naturally homogenizes factors like access to healthcare, economic status, and lifestyle habits [58, 73, 74]. We hypothesize that variations in nutrient access will affect the

3.5 We Are Not Trees but Forests

connectivity of GM and BCA networks, with lower connectivity observed in children with limited consumption of animal proteins and lipids.

Using connectivity in GM and BCA networks using MST as a unifying metric is then a valid proxy for the efficiency of multiscale information transmission within these systems, and hence a good payoff function for assessing the microbiota-gut-brain axis antifragility.

So, on the one hand, we succeeded in identifying a payoff function and now, to complete the antifragility triplet, we only need to define the perturbation.

Assessing the antifragility of the microbiota-gut-brain axis in early age is crucial for understanding its role in shaping lifelong health outcomes, and it is well known that both the gut microbiota ecosystem and brain functioning undergo significant developmental changes during childhood, a period characterized by rapid growth and maturation [44]. The interaction between the host's diet and the gut microbiota during critical developmental windows has profound implications for brain-gut signalling, potentially influencing long-term health and the risk of neurodevelopmental disorders [64, 65]. Early childhood represents a critical period where the ecological dynamics of gut bacteria resemble that of adults, impacting brain development through processes such as synapse elimination and neuronal connectivity formation [66]. Moreover, nutritional factors, particularly those of animal origin like protein and lipids, play a pivotal role in brain structural and functional development during infancy and early childhood [67, 68].

The results of this study [44] the first unifying analysis of brain cortex activity and gut microbiota ecosystem (The system) connectivity (the payoff function) under different levels of protein and lipid intake (perturbation) showing changes of antifragility in the microbiota-gut-brain axis as a whole, due diet differences.

In terms of brain cortex connectivity, the Mutual Information (MI) matrices reveal that the magnitude of relationships between different regions of interest (ROIs) varied depending on protein and lipid intake levels. For example, high protein intake exhibited strongly positive relationships between ROIs. Similarly, most Minimum Spanning Tree (MST) weights, representing structural and functional network connectivity, increased systematically with higher protein intake levels across all classic broadbands, indicating enhanced brain connectivity. Additionally, an increase in MST weight was observed for higher lipid intake levels, albeit to a lesser extent. These findings suggest that adequate protein and lipid intake may contribute to greater brain cortex connectivity, potentially enhancing cognitive function and resilience to perturbations.

In terms of GM, although composition and abundance were not significantly affected by protein or lipid intake levels using standard metrics, when using the new network theory approach, authors do find differences in GM connectivity between intake conditions. Specifically, low protein and lipid intake groups exhibited diminished GM connectivity compared to high intake groups, with MST weight reductions of approximately 50% for both macronutrients. This suggests that inadequate protein and lipid intake levels may compromise GM connectivity, potentially impacting microbiota-gut-brain axis function and antifragility.

Overall, these results highlight the importance of protein and lipid intake in modulating both brain cortex and gut microbiota connectivity, with implications for overall health and resilience in the microbiota-gut-brain axis. Maintaining optimal intake levels of these macronutrients may support robust connectivity within these complex biological networks, enhancing antifragility and adaptive responses to internal and external perturbations.

As a general result, the authors also highlight that assessing the antifragility of the microbiota-gut-brain axis during these formative years is essential for understanding how dietary interventions may influence lifelong health trajectories.

Now consider how contrasting lifestyles between urban traditional communities and modern industrialized cities serve as potent perturbations for the microbiota-gut-brain axis, affecting both internal and external factors. Internally, gut parasites can disrupt physiological processes, including hormonal, neurological, and immunological functions, potentially altering the host's behavior [69–73]. External perturbations arise from sociocultural practices and ecological conditions, particularly impactful during childhood when the gut microbiota is highly sensitive to changes, affecting stability and maturity [74, 75].

The evolutionary influence of different environments and behaviors has shaped human microbiota, with studies comparing industrialized versus non-industrialized populations revealing vulnerabilities to industrialization [78, 79]. Industrialized societies employ strategies such as broad-spectrum antibiotics and ultra-processed foods, which alter gut microbiota diversity and richness [75, 78]. Consequently, individuals in industrialized societies exhibit less diverse microbiota, with taxa losses like Spirochaetes and Prevotellaceae [75, 79].

The shift in micro-ecosystem configuration due to industrialization can adversely affect host health by compromising ecosystem services offered by the gut microbiota, which include immune system regulation, vitamin and hormone synthesis, food digestion, and pathogen protection [80–82]. Assessing microbiota health requires examining ecosystem emergence and self-organization, which are crucial for quantifying current health states and response to perturbations [80–82]. Evaluating internal and external perturbations, such as lifestyle changes or parasites, provides an ecologically valid experiment to determine differences or similarities in gut microbiota criticality/antifragility shaped under these conditions [83].

3.5.4 Social Dimension of the Holobiont

Now, although it is true that "we are not trees but forests", there is a hidden meaning in that sentence, the social dimension of forests that is very clear for humans.

The social dimension of forests emerges from the intricate networks of interactions among various organisms, including trees, plants, fungi, and microorganisms. One of the key aspects of this social dimension is the communication that occurs through mycorrhizal networks, which are symbiotic associations between fungi and plant roots. Mycorrhizal fungi form extensive networks underground, connecting multiple trees and plants within a forest ecosystem.

This mycorrhizal communication not only facilitates the sharing of resources like water, carbon, and nitrogen among plants but also plays a crucial role in shaping the social dynamics of forests. It enables cooperation and mutual support among trees and plants, fostering resilience against environmental stressors and disturbances. Additionally, mycorrhizal networks can contribute to the diversity and stability of forest ecosystems by facilitating the establishment of seedlings and the transfer of beneficial microorganisms.

In this way it turns out to be of great interest to test the social dimension of the microbiota-gut-brain axis, as done by Santoyo and co-workers [58] who re-analyzed existing data [44] to reveal that children living an industrialized urban lifestyle in Mexico City display informational and network characteristics akin to those of parasitized children from a rural indigenous community in the remote mountainous area of Guerrero, México. Consequently, we suggest that during this pivotal stage of gut microbiota development, the industrialized urban lifestyle can be viewed as an external disturbance to the gut microbiota ecosystem. Furthermore, we illustrate that this lifestyle engenders a comparable diminishment in criticality/antifragility, akin to the effects observed with internal perturbations caused by parasitic infection with the helminth A. lumbricoides. Lastly, we discuss various overarching complexity-based strategies aimed at preserving or reinstating the antifragility of the gut ecosystem.

In this social holobiont context, our antifragility triplet ends up being:

System: the gut microbiota ecosystem of children from indigenous marginalized communities in Guerrero state and children from an urban westernized environment in Mexico City.

Payoff function: connectivity of Minimum Spanning Tree of the co-occurrence gut microbiota ecosystem network.

Perturbation: contrasting lifestyles of urban traditional communities Vs modern industrialized cities in terms of diet differences.

The authors analyzed the gut microbiota networks of three distinct populations: Urban (U), Rural Not Parasitized (R-NP), and Rural Parasitized (R-P), employing Graph Edit Distance (GED) analysis to compare their complete network structures. The GED score reflects the dissimilarity between networks, with higher values indicating greater differences. Specifically, the results revealed that both the urban (U) and perturbed rural (R-P) populations exhibited similar effects on gut microbiota networks, suggesting that the urban lifestyle could induce microbiota dysbiosis akin to the perturbed rural environment. This comparison underscores the similarity in perturbation effects between the urban and perturbed rural populations.

Using standard network metrics the authors found that rural populations have greater complexity in terms of the number of nodes and neighbors compared to the urban population. Moreover, the urban microbiota networks exhibited higher heterogeneity, indicative of less complexity compared to rural networks.

Complementary network metrics and differences in Shannon Information (emergence) among the three populations show that both populations under perturbation (R-P and U) displayed significantly lower Shannon information values compared to the unperturbed rural population (R-NP), suggesting reduced microbiota diversity and emergence in perturbed environments.

In general, results suggest that urban lifestyles may lead to microbiota dysbiosis similar to that observed in perturbed rural environments. Additionally, rural populations exhibited greater complexity in their gut microbiota networks compared to urban counterparts, emphasizing the role of contrasting lifestyles in shaping microbiota-gut-brain interactions and antifragility.

Considering the findings of Kaplan et al. [84], which highlight the reduced gut microbiota (GM) diversity in Hispanic populations immigrating to the USA early in life compared to those relocating during adulthood, their research aligns with the emerging concept of the "social microbiome". This emerging concept points out the impact of social and ecological contexts on microbial exchange and, consequently, on the health of GM ecosystems.

By considering the interplay between contrasting lifestyles and GM ecosystems, their study sheds light on the evolution of the Holobiont within specific social contexts, introducing the concept of ecobionts as a novel eco-evolutionary ontological unit [59].

In this regard, their findings reveal significant differences in GM ecosystem antifragility under contrasting lifestyles. Specifically, they observe that urban-industrialized populations exhibit a loss of antifragility akin to that seen in internally perturbed populations, such as those afflicted by parasitosis.

Moreover, their study suggests that the human gut microbiota may have experienced a mass extinction event characterized by the loss of certain species and an increase in others. This phenomenon, coupled with recent lifestyle changes, particularly in diet, has led to profound alterations in the genetic makeup and metabolic processes of the human gut microbiome.

3.6 Implications for Health and Evolutionary Biology

Moving forward, they advocate for a paradigm shift towards an ecological perspective to better understand the role of GM foods in human health. This entails recognizing the dynamic nature of GM ecosystems and their response to perturbations rather than focusing solely on ecosystem integrity.

Finally, their conceptual framework illustrates how path dependence (see Fig. 3.4, in conjunction with different lifestyles, shapes the network structures and responses of GM ecosystems to perturbations. They posit that embracing an antifragility perspective enhances theoretical understanding and holds promise for improving clinical practices and longevity.

3.6 Implications for Health and Evolutionary Biology

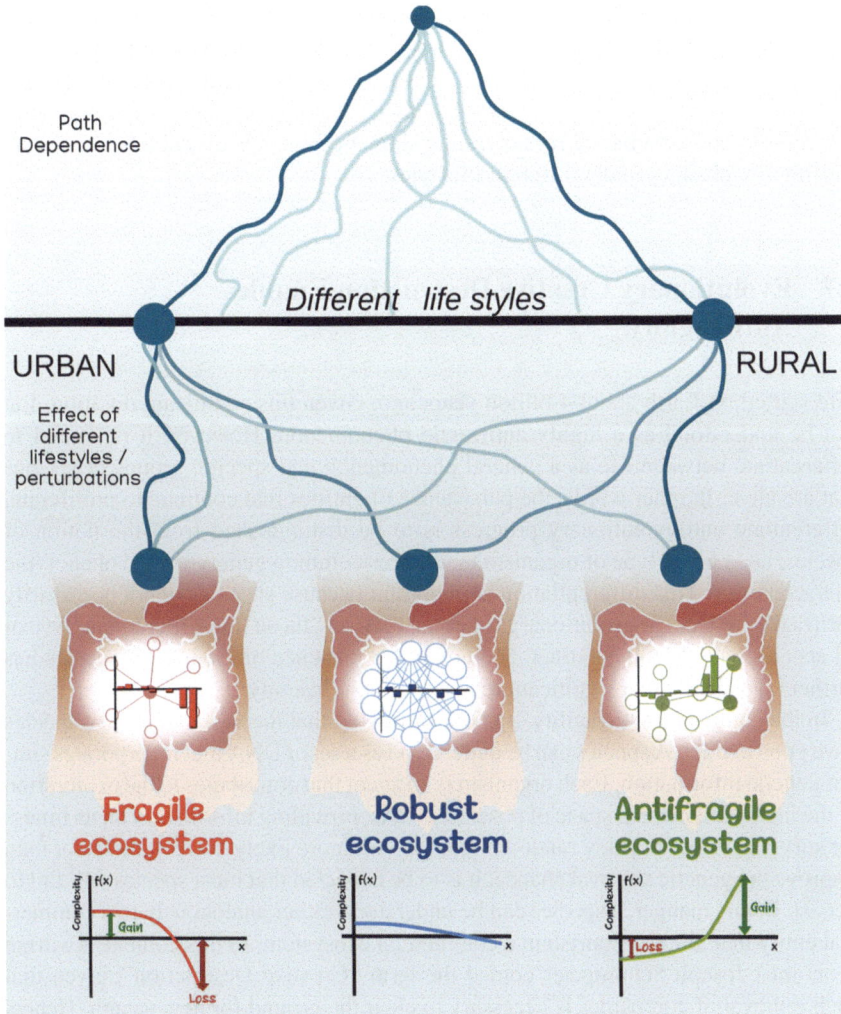

Fig. 3.4 As time goes by, any of three elements of antifragility triplet, the system, the payoff function or the perturbation, may change and those changes chain themselves into a path dependence. In the case of Gut Microbiota, starting at an arbitrary point in time, subsequent lifestyle will change the triplet in such a way that future possible trajectories are conditioned and for the population studied in the case presented, under rural lifestyle the future outcomes tend to be more probably in the robust-antifragile side, meanwhile for urban lifestyle the mus probable future scenarios are on the fragile-robust side. The figure was taken from [58] under the Creative Commons Attribution license

In this sub-chapter, we have shown how the same general framework used for assessing planetary antifragility can be used to study the eco-evolutionary dynamics of holobionts (individuals plus all their symbionts) using a case study of the microbiota-gut-brain axis. We suggest that the holobiont concepts make a good example of how fast (microbiome) and slow (genome) sub-control systems enhance the emergence of antifragile control. We have shown a very interesting proxy for antifragility using network theory, specifically by calculating the connectivity of the minimum spanning tree of the network. Finally, we consider the social holobiont or ecobiont and summarise recent results showing how gut microbiota ecosystem antifragility changes under different lifestyles.

3.7 Evolutionary Creative Destruction Enables Antifragility

Life started on Earth about 4 billion years ago. Given this significant duration, life can be understood as a highly antifragile phenomenon. However, it is crucial to differentiate between life as a general phenomenon and specific groups or species that are alive. In other words, the persistence of entities that continue to proliferate, differentiate and evolutionary progress is to be distinguished from the notion of species, i.e. a given type of organism that shares common genotypic and phenotypic characteristics. This differentiation is important because species are not necessarily antifragile, at least in evolutionary timescales. Along those lines, more than 99% of all species have become extinct. Moreover, the presence of the human species has further contributed to a significant reduction of biodiversity.

In the context of antifragility, it is not surprising that the vast majority of species have gone extinct. A species can be understood as a set of DNA that incorporates similar genetic information. Each organism is an agent that contributes to the exploration of the high-dimensional space of possible DNAs, providing information on its fitness for survival. Given that any random mutation will more likely deteriorate rather than improve the genetic survival chance, it is to be expected that most species will fail to persist. In this manner, a species can be understood rather analogously to a commercial entity that aims to flourish in a commercial ecosystem. In this context, Austrian economist Joseph Schumpeter coined the term "Creative Destruction", given that such removal of companies is necessary to clear the ground for new wealth. Hence, the framework of antifragility offers an attractive conceptual basis for understanding the existence of destruction in nature as a necessary component of evolution and progression.

Notably, this analogy can be seen in other domains of natural development. Along those lines, the study of [60] presents a computational model for neocortical development. Following experimental data, it reproduces a significant proportion of cell death during normal development. This aligns with the concept of antifragility, which is usually the global result of multiple interacting local components: many more neurons are born since it is likely that many won't end up at the correct locations or the correct proportions of cell types. Only when the neuronal locations and the population sizes are well-suited is the neuronal architecture appropriate to perform its function. Since the brain is organized in a modular fashion, with specialised areas dealing with pertinent tasks, different brain regions will require different architectures. Cell death is a powerful ingredient in neurodevelopment that allows control of architectural development. To this end, our work [60] supports these hypotheses using a mechanistic modelling approach called agent-based modelling [61]. Moreover, the study also demonstrates surprising correspondance to pathologies observed in certain neurodevelopmental disorders such as polymicrogyria or autistic spectrum disorders.

Overall, the observed occurrence of death, both on the level of individual cells as well as species, points towards evolutionary advantages concerning robustness and antifragility. This has intriguing implications also for human methodologies in terms of creating systems or synthetic networks that are prone to face challenges, e.g. power networks or supply chains. We suggest that an evolving approach where individual elements are frequently removed and new elements are added could provide a fruitful approach for generating adaptive systems that express antifragility.

Acknowledgments We acknowledge the contribution of Mrs. Elvia Ramírez-Carrillo from Universidad Nacional Autónoma de México and Mr. Ari Barnett from the Moffitt Cancer Center & University of South Florida in writing this chapter.

References

1. Cristian Axenie, Oliver López-Corona, Michail A Makridis, Meisam Akbarzadeh, Matteo Saveriano, Alexandru Stancu, and Jeffrey West. Antifragility in complex dynamical systems. *npj Complexity*, 1(1):12, 2024.
2. J Martin Bland and Douglas G Altman. Survival probabilities (the Kaplan-Meier method). *BMJ*, 317(7172):1572–1580, 1998.
3. Haeun Hwangbo, Sarah C. Patterson, Andy Dai, Deborah Plana, and Adam C. Palmer. Additivity predicts the efficacy of most approved combination therapies for advanced cancer. *Nature Cancer*, 4(12):1693–1704, 2023.
4. Sarah C Patterson, Amy E Pomeroy, and Adam C Palmer. Ultrasensitive response explains the benefit of combination chemotherapy despite drug antagonism. *Molecular Cancer Therapeutics*, pages OF1–OF15, 2024.
5. Robert A Gatenby, Ariosto S Silva, Robert J Gillies, and B Roy Frieden. Adaptive therapy. *Cancer Research*, 69(11):4894–4903, 2009.
6. Jessica J. Cunningham, Joel S. Brown, Robert A. Gatenby, and Katerina Stankova. Optimal control to develop therapeutic strategies for metastatic castrate resistant prostate cancer. *Journal of Theoretical Biology*, 459:67–78, 2018.
7. Elsa Hansen and Andrew F. Read. Cancer therapy: Attempt cure or manage drug resistance? *Evolutionary Applications*, 13(7):1660–1672, 2020.
8. Jeffrey West, Yongqian Ma, and Paul K Newton. Capitalizing on competition: An evolutionary model of competitive release in metastatic castration resistant prostate cancer treatment. *Journal of Theoretical Biology*, 455:249–260, 2018.
9. Jeffrey West, Jill Gallaher, Maximilian Strobl, Mark Robertson-Tessi, and Alexander R.A. Anderson. The fundamentals of evolutionary therapy in cancer. In *Cancer Systems Biology and Translational Mathematical Oncology*. Oxford University Press, 2023.
10. Austin P.H. Dove, Anthony Cmelak, Kaleb Darrow, Kyra N. McComas, Mudit Chowdhary, Jason Beckta, and Austin N. Kirschner. The use of low-dose radiation therapy in osteoarthritis:

A review. *International Journal of Radiation Oncology*Biology*Physics*, 114(2):203–220, October 2022.
11. R Mücke, O Micke, MH Seegenschmiedt, and U Schäfer. Leitlinen in der strahlentherapie: Strahlentherapie gutartiger erkrankungen–fachgruppenspezifische evidenzbasierte s2e-leitlinie der deutschen gesellschaft für radioonkologie (degro), 2018.
12. Beatriz Alvarez, Angel Montero, Ovidio Hernando, Raquel Ciervide, Juan Garcia, Mercedes Lopez, Mariola Garcia-Aranda, Xin Chen, Ines Flores, Emilio Sanchez, et al. Radiotherapy ct-based contouring atlas for non-malignant skeletal and soft tissue disorders: a practical proposal from spanish experience. *The British Journal of Radiology*, 94(1124):20200809, 2021.
13. G. Hildebrandt, M. P. Seed, C. N. Freemantle, C. A. S. Alam, P. R. Colville-Nash, and K. R. Trott. Mechanisms of the anti-inflammatory activity of low-dose radiation therapy. *International Journal of Radiation Biology*, 74(3):367–378, 1998.
14. Jeffrey West, Bina Desai, Maximilian Strobl, Luke Pierik, Robert Vander Velde, Cole Armagost, Richard Miles, Mark Robertson-Tessi, Andriy Marusyk, and Alexander RA Anderson. Antifragile therapy. *BioRxiv*, pages 2020–10, 2020.
15. Luke Pierik, Patricia McDonald, Alexander RA Anderson, and Jeffrey West. Second-order effects of chemotherapy pharmacodynamics and pharmacokinetics on tumor regression and cachexia. *Bulletin of Mathematical Biology*, 86(5):47, 2024.
16. Nassim Nicholas Taleb and Jeffrey West. Working with convex responses: Antifragility from finance to oncology. *Entropy*, 25(2):343, 2023.
17. Christopher M. Baker, Matthew J. Ferrari, and Katriona Shea. Beyond dose: Pulsed antibiotic treatment schedules can maintain individual benefit while reducing resistance. *Scientific Reports*, 8(1), April 2018.
18. Elsa Hansen, Jason Karslake, Robert J. Woods, Andrew F. Read, and Kevin B. Wood. Antibiotics can be used to contain drug-resistant bacteria by maintaining sufficiently large sensitive populations. *PLOS Biology*, 18(5):e3000713, 2020.
19. Jessica J. Cunningham. A call for integrated metastatic management. *Nature Ecology & Evolution*, 3(7):996–998, 2019.
20. Jingsong Zhang, Jessica Cunningham, Joel Brown, and Robert Gatenby. Evolution-based mathematical models significantly prolong response to abiraterone in metastatic castrate-resistant prostate cancer and identify strategies to further improve outcomes. *Elife*, 11:e76284, 2022.
21. Peter Bayer and Jeffrey West. Games and the treatment convexity of cancer. *Dynamic Games and Applications*, 13(4):1088–1105, 2023.
22. Maximilian AR Strobl, Alexandra L Martin, Jeffrey West, Jill Gallaher, Mark Robertson-Tessi, Robert Gatenby, Robert Wenham, Philip K Maini, Mehdi Damaghi, and Alexander RA Anderson. To modulate or to skip: De-escalating parp inhibitor maintenance therapy in ovarian cancer using adaptive therapy. *Cell Systems*, 15(6):510–525, 2024.
23. Huitzil, S., Huepe, C., Aldana, M., and Frank, A. (2023). The missing link: how the holobiont concept provides a genetic framework for rapid evolution and the inheritance of acquired characteristics. *Frontiers in Ecology and Evolution*, 11, 1279938.
24. Huitzil, S., Sandoval-Motta, S., Frank, A., and Aldana, M. (2020). Phenotype heritability in holobionts: An evolutionary model, in *Symbiosis: Cellular, Molecular, Medical and Evolutionary Aspects*, Cham: Springer.
25. Huitzil, S., Sandoval-Motta, S., Frank, A., and Aldana, M. (2018). Modeling the role of the microbiome in evolution, *Front. Physiol.*, **9**, 1836. https://doi.org/10.3389/fphys.2018.01836
26. Cox, G. W. (2004). *Alien species and evolution: the evolutionary ecology of exotic plants, animals, microbes, and interacting native species*. Washington, DC: Island Press.
27. Brucker, R. M., and Bordenstein, S. R. (2012). Speciation by symbiosis, *Trends Ecol. Evol.*, **27**, 443–451. https://doi.org/10.1016/j.tree.2012.03.011
28. Rudman, S. M., Greenblum, S., Hughes, R. C., Rajpurohit, S., Kiratli, O., Lowder, D. B., et al. (2019). Microbiome composition shapes rapid genomic adaptation of *Drosophila melanogaster*, *Proc. Natl. Acad. Sci.*, **116**, 20025–20032. https://doi.org/10.1073/pnas.1907787116

References

29. Kolodny, O., and Schulenburg, H. (2020). Microbiome-mediated plasticity directs host evolution along several distinct time scales, *Philos. Trans. R. Soc. B*, **375**, 20190589. https://doi.org/10.1098/rstb.2019.0589
30. Sharon, G., Segal, D., Ringo, J. M., Hefetz, A., Zilber-Rosenberg, I., and Rosenberg, E. (2010). Commensal bacteria play a role in mating preference of *Drosophila melanogaster*, *Proc. Natl. Acad. Sci.*, **107**, 20051–20056. https://doi.org/10.1073/pnas.1009906107
31. Foster, K. R., Schluter, J., Coyte, K. Z., and Rakoff-Nahoum, S. (2017). The evolution of the host microbiome as an ecosystem on a leash. *Nature*, **548**, 43–51. https://doi.org/10.1038/nature23292
32. Collens, A., Kelley, E., and Katz, L. A. (2019). The concept of the hologenome, an epigenetic phenomenon, challenges aspects of the modern evolutionary synthesis. *Journal of Experimental Zoology Part B: Molecular and Developmental Evolution*, **332**, 349–355. https://doi.org/10.1002/jez.b.22915
33. Veigl, S., Suárez, J., and Stencel, A. (2019). Does inheritance need a rethink? Conceptual tools to extend inheritance beyond DNA. *Extended Evolutionary Synthesis*.
34. Henry, L. P., Bruijning, M., Forsberg, S. K., and Ayroles, J. F. (2021). The microbiome extends host evolutionary potential. *Front. Ecol. Evol.*, **9**, 649424. https://doi.org/10.3389/fevo.2021.649424
35. Ashe, A., Colot, V., and Oldroyd, B. P. (2021). How does epigenetics influence the course of evolution? *Philos. Trans. R. Soc. Lond. B Biol. Sci.*, **376**(1826), 20200111. https://doi.org/10.1098/rstb.2020.0111
36. Sandoval-Motta, S., Aldana, M., and Frank, A. (2017). Evolving ecosystems: Inheritance and selection in the light of the microbiome. *Arch. Med. Res.*, **48**, 780–789. https://doi.org/10.1016/j.arcmed.2018.01.002
37. Tan, J., Kerstetter, J. E., and Turcotte, M. M. (2021). Eco-evolutionary interaction between microbiome presence and rapid biofilm evolution determines plant host fitness. *Nat. Ecol. Evol.*, **5**, 670–676. https://doi.org/10.1038/s41559-021-01406-2
38. Moeller, A. H., Li, Y., Mpoudi Ngole, E., Ahuka-Mundeke, S., Lonsdorf, E. V., Pusey, A. E., et al. (2014). Rapid changes in the gut microbiome during human evolution. *Proc. Natl. Acad. Sci.*, **111**, 16431–16435. https://doi.org/10.1073/pnas.1419136111
39. Howells, E., Beltran, V., Larsen, N., Bay, L., Willis, B., and Van Oppen, M. (2012). Coral thermal tolerance shaped by local adaptation of photosymbionts. *Nat. Climate Change*, **2**, 116–120. https://doi.org/10.1038/nclimate1330
40. Baldo, L., Pretus, J. L., Riera, J. L., Musilova, Z., Bitja Nyom, A. R., and Salzburger, W. (2017). Convergence of gut microbiotas in the adaptive radiations of African cichlid fishes. *ISME J.*, **11**, 1975–1987. https://doi.org/10.1038/ismej.2017.62
41. King, K. C., Brockhurst, M. A., Vasieva, O., Paterson, S., Betts, A., Ford, S. A., et al. (2016). Rapid evolution of microbe-mediated protection against pathogens in a worm host. *ISME J.*, **10**, 1915–1924. https://doi.org/10.1038/ismej.2015.259
42. Chen, D. W., and Garud, N. R. (2022). Rapid evolution and strain turnover in the infant gut microbiome. *Genome Res.*, **32**, 1124–1136. https://doi.org/10.1101/gr.276306.121
43. Moran, N. A., and Yun, Y. (2015). Experimental replacement of an obligate insect symbiont. *Proc. Natl. Acad. Sci.*, **112**, 2093–2096. https://doi.org/10.1073/pnas.1420037112
44. Ramírez-Carrillo, E., G-Santoyo, I., López-Corona, O., Rojas-Ramos, O. A., Falcón, L. I., Gaona, O., ... and Nieto, J. (2023). Similar connectivity of gut microbiota and brain activity networks is mediated by animal protein and lipid intake in children from a Mexican indigenous population. *PLoS One*, **18**(6), e0281385.
45. Rosenberg, E., Koren, O., Reshef, L., Efrony, R., and Zilber-Rosenberg, I. (2007). The role of microorganisms in coral health, disease and evolution. *Nature Reviews Microbiology*, **5**, 355–362. https://doi.org/10.1038/nrmicro1635
46. Rosenberg, E., Sharon, G., and Zilber-Rosenberg, I. (2009). The hologenome theory of evolution contains Lamarckian aspects within a Darwinian framework. *Environ. Microbiol.*, **11**, 2959–2962. https://doi.org/10.1111/j.1462-2920.2009.01995.x

47. Rosenberg, E., and Zilber-Rosenberg, I. (2016). Microbes drive evolution of animals and plants: the hologenome concept. *MBio*, **7**, e01395–15. https://doi.org/10.1128/mBio.01395-15
48. Daisy W Chen and Nandita R Garud. "Rapid evolution and strain turnover in the infant gut microbiome." *Genome Research*, 32(6):1124–1136, 2022. Cold Spring Harbor Laboratory.
49. Andrew H Moeller, Yingying Li, Eitel Mpoudi Ngole, Steve Ahuka-Mundeke, Elizabeth V Lonsdorf, Anne E Pusey, Martine Peeters, Beatrice H Hahn, and Howard Ochman. "Rapid changes in the gut microbiome during human evolution." *Proceedings of the National Academy of Sciences*, 111(46):16431–16435, 2014. National Academy of Sciences.
50. Emily J Howells, VH Beltran, NW Larsen, LK Bay, BL Willis, and MJH Van Oppen. "Coral thermal tolerance shaped by local adaptation of photosymbionts." *Nature Climate Change*, 2(2):116–120, 2012. Nature Publishing Group UK London.
51. Laura Baldo, Joan Lluís Pretus, Joan Lluís Riera, Zuzana Musilova, Arnold Roger Bitja Nyom, and Walter Salzburger. "Convergence of gut microbiotas in the adaptive radiations of African cichlid fishes." *The ISME journal*, 11(9):1975–1987, 2017. Oxford University Press.
52. King, K. C., Brockhurst, M. A., Vasieva, O., Paterson, S., Betts, A., Ford, S. A., et al. (2016). Rapid evolution of microbe-mediated protection against pathogens in a worm host. *ISME J*, 10, 1915–1924. https://doi.org/10.1038/ismej.2015.259
53. Moran, N. A., & Yun, Y. (2015). Experimental replacement of an obligate insect symbiont. *Proc. Natl. Acad. Sci.*, 112, 2093–2096. https://doi.org/10.1073/pnas.1420037112
54. Moran, N. A. (2007). Symbiosis as an adaptive process and source of phenotypic complexity. *Proc. Natl. Acad. Sci.*, 104, 8627–8633. https://doi.org/10.1073/pnas.0611659104
55. Danchin, É., Charmantier, A., Champagne, F. A., Mesoudi, A., Pujol, B., and Blanchet, S. (2011). Beyond DNA: integrating inclusive inheritance into an extended theory of evolution, *Nat. Rev. Genet.*, **12**, 475–486. https://doi.org/10.1038/nrg3028
56. Pflughoeft, K. J., & Versalovic, J. (2012). Human microbiome in health and disease. *Annual Review of Pathology: Mechanisms of Disease*, 7, 99–122. https://doi.org/10.1146/annurev-pathol-011811-132421
57. Shreiner, A. B., Kao, J. Y., & Young, V. B. (2015). The gut microbiome in health and in disease. *Current Opinion in Gastroenterology*, 31, 69. https://doi.org/10.1097/MOG.0000000000000139
58. Isaac, G-Santoyo, Ramírez-Carrillo, E., Sanchez, J. D., and López-Corona, O. (2023). Potential long consequences from internal and external ecology: loss of gut microbiota antifragility in children from an industrialized population compared with an indigenous rural lifestyle. *Journal of Developmental Origins of Health and Disease*, **14**(4), 469-480.
59. López-Corona, O., Ramírez-Carrillo, E., and Magallanes, G. (2019). The rise of the technobionts: toward a new ontology to understand current planetary crisis. *Researchers.One*. https://researchers.one/articles/19.01.00001v1
60. Bauer, R., Clowry, G. & Kaiser, M. Creative destruction: a basic computational model of cortical layer formation. *Cerebral Cortex*. **31**, 3237–3253 (2021).
61. Breitwieser, L., Hesam, A., De Montigny, J., Vavourakis, V., Iosif, A., Jennings, J., Kaiser, M., Manca, M., Di Meglio, A., Al-Ars, Z. & Others BioDynaMo: a modular platform for high-performance agent-based simulation. *Bioinformatics*. **38**, 453–460 (2022).
62. Saba, V., Premi, E., Cristillo, V., Gazzina, S., Palluzzi, F., Zanetti, O., Gasparotti, R., Padovani, A., Borroni, B. & Grassi, M. Brain connectivity and information-flow breakdown revealed by a minimum spanning tree-based analysis of MRI data in behavioral variant frontotemporal dementia. *Frontiers In Neuroscience*. **13** pp. 211 (2019).
63. Mayer, E. A. (2011). Gut feelings: The emerging biology of gut-brain communication. Nature Reviews Neuroscience, 12(8), 453–466. [Nature Publishing Group UK London].
64. De Filippo, C., Cavalieri, D., Di Paola, M., Ramazzotti, M., Poullet, J. B., Massart, S., Collini, S., Pieraccini, G., & Lionetti, P. (2010). Impact of diet in shaping gut microbiota revealed by a comparative study in children from Europe and rural Africa. *Proceedings of the National Academy of Sciences*, 107(33), 14691-14696. National Acad Sciences.
65. Sandhu, K. V., Sherwin, E., Schellekens, H., Stanton, C., Dinan, T. G., & Cryan, J. F. (2017). Feeding the microbiota-gut-brain axis: diet, microbiome, and neuropsychiatry. *Translational Research*, 179, 223–244. Elsevier.

References

66. Paus, T., Keshavan, M., & Giedd, J. N. (2008). Why do many psychiatric disorders emerge during adolescence? *Nature Reviews Neuroscience*, *9*(12), 947-957. Nature Publishing Group UK London.
67. Duerden, E. G., Thompson, B., Poppe, T., Alsweiler, J., Gamble, G., Jiang, Y., Leung, M., Tottman, A. C., Wouldes, T., Miller, S. P., et al. (2021). Early protein intake predicts functional connectivity and neurocognition in preterm born children. *Scientific Reports*, *11*(1), 4085. Nature Publishing Group UK London.
68. Benton, D. (2010). The influence of dietary status on the cognitive performance of children. *Molecular Nutrition & Food Research*, *54*(4), 457–470. Wiley Online Library.
69. Romano, M. C., Jiménez, P., Miranda-Brito, C., & Valdez, R. A. (2015). Parasites and steroid hormones: corticosteroid and sex steroid synthesis, their role in the parasite physiology and development. *Frontiers in Neuroscience*, *9*, 224. Frontiers Media SA.
70. Johnson, T. P., & Nath, A. (2018). Neurological syndromes driven by postinfectious processes or unrecognized persistent infections. *Current Opinion in Neurology*, *31*(3), 318–324. LWW.
71. Shepherd, C., Navarro, S., Wangchuk, P., Wilson, D., Daly, N. L., & Loukas, A. (2015). Identifying the immunomodulatory components of helminths. *Parasite Immunology*, *37*(6), 293–303. Wiley Online Library.
72. Adamo, S. A. (2002). Modulating the modulators: parasites, neuromodulators and host behavioral change. *Brain Behavior and Evolution*, *60*(6), 370–377. S. Karger AG.
73. González-Tokman, D., Córdoba-Aguilar, A., González-Santoyo, I., & Lanz-Mendoza, H. (2011). Infection effects on feeding and territorial behaviour in a predatory insect in the wild. *Animal Behaviour*, *81*(6), 1185–1194. Elsevier.
74. Olm, M. R., Dahan, D., Carter, M. M., Merrill, B. D., Yu, F. B., Jain, S., Meng, X., Tripathi, S., Wastyk, H., Neff, N., et al. (2022). Robust variation in infant gut microbiome assembly across a spectrum of lifestyles. *Science*, *376*(6598), 1220–1223. American Association for the Advancement of Science.
75. Sonnenburg, J. L.,& Sonnenburg, E. D. (2019). Vulnerability of the industrialized microbiota. *Science*, *366*(6464), eaaw9255. American Association for the Advancement of Science.
76. Gammaitoni, L., Hänggi, P., Jung, P. & Marchesoni, F. Stochastic resonance. *Reviews Of Modern Physics*. **70**, 223 (1998).
77. Baker, S. & Chapin, F. Going beyond "it depends:" the role of context in shaping participation in natural resource management. *Ecology And Society*. **23** (2018).
78. Rosas-Plaza, S., Hernández-Terán, A., Navarro-Díaz, M., Escalante, A. E., Morales-Espinosa, R.,& Cerritos, R. (2022). Human gut microbiome across different lifestyles: from hunter-gatherers to urban populations. *Frontiers in Microbiology*, *13*, 843170. Frontiers.
79. Sánchez-Quinto, A., Cerqueda-García, D., Falcón, L. I., Gaona, O., Martínez-Correa, S., Nieto, J.,& G-Santoyo, I. (2020). Gut microbiome in children from indigenous and urban communities in México: Different subsistence models, different microbiomes. *Microorganisms*, *8*(10), 1592. MDPI.
80. Kapasi, A. J., Dittrich, S., González, I. J., & Rodwell, T. C. (2016). Host biomarkers for distinguishing bacterial from non-bacterial causes of acute febrile illness: a comprehensive review. *PloS One*, *11*(8), e0160278. Public Library of Science San Francisco, CA USA.
81. Ding, R.-X., Goh, W.-R., Wu, R.-N., Yue, X.-Q., Luo, X., Khine, W. W. T., Wu, J.-R., & Lee, Y.-K. (2019). Revisit gut microbiota and its impact on human health and disease. *Journal of Food and Drug Analysis*, *27*(3), 623–631. Elsevier.
82. Ramírez-Carrillo, E., Gaona, O., Nieto, J., Sánchez-Quinto, A., Cerqueda-García, D., Falcón, L. I., Rojas-Ramos, O. A., & González-Santoyo, I. (2020). Disturbance in human gut microbiota networks by parasites and its implications in the incidence of depression. *Scientific Reports*, *10*(1), 3680. Nature Publishing Group UK London.
83. Kim, P.-J., & Price, N. D. (2011). Genetic co-occurrence network across sequenced microbes. *PLoS Computational Biology*, *7*(12), e1002340. Public Library of Science San Francisco, USA.
84. Kaplan, R. C., Wang, Z., Usyk, M., Sotres-Alvarez, D., Daviglus, M. L., Schneiderman, N., Talavera, G. A., Gellman, M. D., Thyagarajan, B., Moon, J.-Y., et al. (2019). Gut microbiome composition in the Hispanic Community Health Study/Study of Latinos is shaped by geographic relocation, environmental factors, and obesity. *Genome Biology*, *20*, 1–21. Springer.

Chapter 4
Interventional Antifragility

Abstract This chapter introduces interventional antifragility as the externally-driven reaching dynamics of a natural dynamic system. It describes the benefit derived from input distribution unevenness, based on the emergent system dynamics in a closed loop with a signal driving the system behavior towards prescribed dynamics. We consider methods for the detection, analysis, modelling, and control of cancer therapy and neural disease systems antifragility.

4.1 Defining Interventional Antifragility

The previous chapters have illustrated the connection between the convexity of the payoff function, $f(x)$, and the outcome benefit to input variation, with or without external noise and disturbances. In this chapter, we turn our attention to the design and implementation of controllers to intervene and perturb the system. The control-theoretic approach to antifragility utilizes timescale separation and redundant overcompensation with variable structure control, as described in the sections below.

4.2 Closed-Loop Antifragility in Tumor-Immune-Drug Dynamics

This sub-chapter examines the potential for modifying a complex system's dynamics by implementing a closed-loop antifragile control mechanism. The efficacy of therapeutic intervention is contingent upon the tumor's response to treatment, which is influenced by many factors, including the severity of the disease and the strength of the patient's immune response. The gold standard cancer therapies are, in the majority of cases, fragile when attempting to achieve a balance between tumor-kill ratio and patient toxicity. Recent research has demonstrated that cancer therapy can be optimized when addressing adaptive drug resistance and immune escape patterns developed by evolving tumors. This is attributable to the stochastic and volatile nature of the interactions at the tumor environment level, tissue vasculature, and immune landscape induced by drugs.

In this section, we examine the route towards antifragile therapy control, which entails the development of treatment plans that are not merely robust but exceed the boundaries of robustness. In more detail, we present the initial application of a control-theoretic approach to enable therapeutic protocols to accommodate the systemic variability in tumor-immune-drug interactions, thereby enhancing tumor destruction with reduced patient toxicity. In light of the anti-symmetric interactions within a model of the tumor-immune-drug network, we introduce the antifragile control framework, which demonstrates promising results in the simulation of clinical treatment design.

4.2.1 Problem Statement

The objective of therapeutic intervention is to induce deliberate and regulated alterations in the tumor microenvironment through the precise timing and dosage of the administered pharmacological agents. Nevertheless, such an intervention results in significant disruptions to the tumor's evolution and environment, as well as the structure of surrounding normal cells, vasculature and, naturally, the immune system response [12]. Given the stochastic and complex nature of such processes, therapeutic schemes tend to be unsuccessful in the face of the systemic variability and volatility of the effects they have upon the tumor. In other words, they are vulnerable. It is typically the objective of such therapies to adhere to precise and fixed schedules, as devised by clinicians, to control both the administration time and the dose magnitude and to obtain a targeted response while minimizing toxicity. However, the stochastic and patient-specific nature of tumor-immune-drug dynamics presents a significant challenge to the development of suitable patient-centred interventions.

In light of the encouraging preliminary outcomes of the antifragile therapy, we put forth the proposition of developing an adaptive antifragile therapy. This approach would entail making treatment adjustments to regulate tumor growth and manage toxicity based on tumor response to ensure clinical feasibility and beneficial outcomes. The approach proposed by West et al. [16] allows for a straightforward prediction of optimal dose treatments for a wide range of treatment schedules that result in the same cumulative drug dose. However, our work will go beyond this by enabling a control-theoretic framework that can validate the link between the shape of the dose-response curve and the treatment schedule. In more precise terms, our objective is to construct a framework for the dosing and scheduling of treatments that can drive the dynamics of the tumor-immune-drug network towards a patient-specific shape of dose-response.

4.2.2 Closed-Loop Interventions in Cancer Therapy

Cancer therapies follow national or international guidelines that typically outline the recommendations from the latest and most successful research studies on cumulative dosing, therapy staging, and therapy combinations. However, the therapy parameters, such as dose frequency and dose magnitude, are typically based on the prescribing physician's assessment of the specific tumor characteristics (i.e., BRCA1 and BRCA2 gene mutations in breast cancer for instance) and behavior (i.e., multistage carcinogenesis, from tumor genesis to metastasis).

The optimisation of chemotherapy strategies to achieve an optimal efficacy/toxicity ratio can be achieved by exploiting the nonlinear tumor response dynamics and adaptive control of dosage under patient-specific tumor–immune–drug interactions. However, the intricate dynamics that govern patient-specific tumor-immune-drug interactions are characterized by a high degree of variability, volatility and randomness. Control theory provides a systematic framework for addressing such a landscape, ensuring not merely tolerating systemic variability but also capitalizing on it. This behavior is captured by the recently developed antifragile therapy paradigm, as outlined in [16]. Rather than focusing on antifragility theory and heuristics to inform treatment scheduling or resistance management plans, we propose a systematic approach to building chemotherapy control systems that are antifragile.

This sub-section provides system design "recipes" and establishes the basis for a novel framework for designing control systems that can operate in the presence of the randomness, variability, and volatility of the patient-specific tumor–immune–drug dynamics.

4.2.3 Tumor–Immune–Drug Network Model

To analyze and evaluate the antifragile control framework, we employ a network model that captures the tumor–immune–drug interactions from [22], which is further refined with the parametrization suggested in [23, 24]. The original model comprises three populations of cells (i.e., tumor, immune and normal cells) which evolve through mutual connections and in response to the presence or absence of the chemotherapeutic drug. The network model used in this study is depicted in Fig. 4.1.

The ordinary differential equations (ODE) describing the dynamics of the tumor–immune–drug network are introduced in Eqs. (4.1)–(4.4). The network interaction model captures competition (i.e., c_1, c_2, c_3, c_4 parameters) and modulation among tumor and immune and normal cells (i.e., ρ, α, d_1 parameters, as well as the cooperation within each of the three populations (i.e., s, r_1, r_2 parameters), accounting for a basic form of self-excitation. The drug acts upon all three cell populations in the network model by killing cells with a certain rate (i.e., a_1, a_2, a_3 parameters), as shown in the mapping in Fig. 4.1-right panel. As illustrated in the network model,

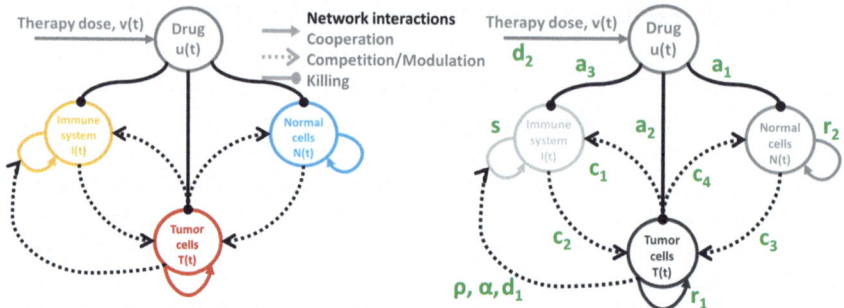

Fig. 4.1 Network model of tumor–immune–drug interactions. Left panel: population cell interactions; Right panel: differential equations parameters mapped on the network populations interactions

the presence of tumor cells elicits an immune response, as evidenced by the positive nonlinear growth term $\frac{\rho I(t) T(t)}{\alpha + T(t)}$ within the immune evolution in Eqs. (4.1)–(4.4).

$$\frac{dN(t)}{dt} = r_2 N(t)(1 - b_2 N(t)) - c_4 T(t) N(t) - a_1 (1 - e^{u(t)}) N(t) \tag{4.1}$$

$$\frac{dT(t)}{dt} = r_1 T(t)(1 - b_1 T(t)) - c_2 T(t) I(t) - c_3 T(t) N(t) - a_2 (1 - e^{u(t)}) T(t) \tag{4.2}$$

$$\frac{dI(t)}{dt} = s + \frac{\rho I(t) T(t)}{\alpha + T(t)} - c_1 I(t) T(t) - d_1 I(t) - a_3 (1 - e^{u(t)}) I(t) \tag{4.3}$$

$$\frac{du(t)}{dt} = v(t) - d_2 u(t) \tag{4.4}$$

4.2.3.1 Drug-Free Evolution

This sub-section presents the drug-free evolution of the model, which will facilitate the subsequent analysis and control design. To analyze the basic dynamics of the tumor–immune–drug network model, we consider the cumulative drug dose $u(t) = v(t) = 0$ when simulating the ODEs of the system. We start with a relatively large tumor burden $T(0) = 0.25$ and an analysis period of $t = 150$ days (i.e., a typical duration of a chemotherapy schema). The initial tumor size corresponds to a tumor with approximately 0.20×10^{11} cells, or, in other words, a solid tumor of radius between 1.8 and 3.9 cm. To provide the reader with some reference, the clinical detection threshold for a solid tumor is typically around 10^7 cells, this sets our chosen initial tumor volume of 0.20×10^{11} above the clinical detection level. We also consider a patient with a weak immune system (but above the level of an immune-compromised patient) $I(0) = 0.1$. The immune threshold rate α is chosen inversely related to the immune response curve such that when the number of tumor cells T

4.2 Closed-Loop Antifragility in Tumor-Immune-Drug Dynamics

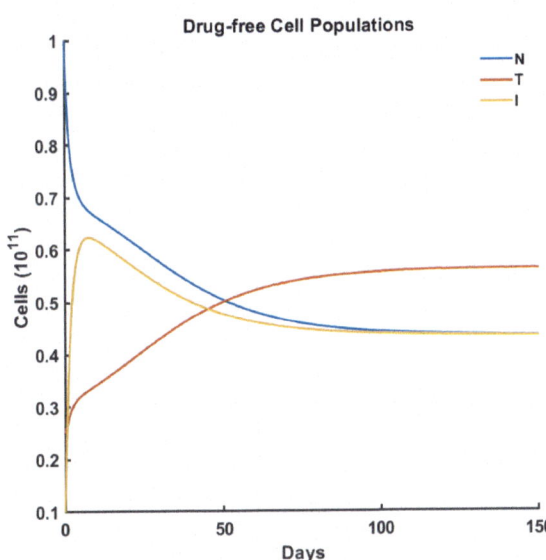

Fig. 4.2 Drug-free evolution of the network model. The immune system (I) reacts by proliferating T-cells when the tumor (T) population (and tumor itself) reaches a threshold triggering immune-surveillance. The normal cells (N) production decreases as the tumor expands. In this case, without any drug administration, the tumor proliferates uncontrollably, escaping immune surveillance

is equal to α, the immune response rate is at half of its maximum. To guide our control-theoretic design of therapy, we perform the null-space analysis of the drug-free dynamics. The evolution of each of the three interacting cell populations is depicted in Fig. 4.2.

As we see in Fig. 4.2, once the tumor has a considerable size (i.e., $T(0) = 0.20$), the immune system reacts with a very steep rise time in the first 10 days. The immune response is then modulated by the tumor proliferation and the decay in normal cell production, which we see already after 50 days.

We offer the reader the possibility to reproduce the analysis and reuse the models (i.e., tumor–immune–drug and control theoretic models) from the experiments performed in this study by downloading the code available on GitLab.[1]

4.2.4 Interventional Antifragility Control

This section presents a detailed account of the mathematical apparatus of antifragile control, encompassing a comprehensive overview of the underlying theory and principles, as well as a systematic exposition of the synthesis of control.

When examining control systems, inducing such behavior in a feedback control loop represents a novel approach to design and synthesis. (1) Redundant overcompensation can result in the system entering an overshooting mode, thereby building additional capacity and resilience in anticipation; (2) Structure variability can induce

---

[1] Code available at: https://gitlab.com/akii-microlab/antifragile-therapy-ctrl.

stressors and convey inherent information that emerges only under conditions of volatility and randomness. The alteration of system dynamics resulting from the application of a high-frequency switching control signal; and (3) the implementation of high-frequency control activity in opposition to a "tight control" approach, which merely eliminates the advantageous impact of noise and volatility within the closed-loop dynamics. This section will provide an overview of the aforementioned concepts and their practical applications in the context of therapy control.

The objective of antifragile control is to identify and capitalize on the relationships between the nonlinearity of drug dose-response and the characteristics of the outcomes (e.g., tumor kill ratio, toxicity ratio and their mean and variability) within the context of complex tumor–immune–drug dynamics. However, a key challenge remains in quantifying antifragility.

As shown in the previous section, the shape of the drug dose–response is a useful heuristic to detect antifragility and, implicitly, inform tumor evolution and optimal dosing plans within a therapy schedule. Yet, assessing the drug dose–response in complex tumor–immune–drug models, such as the one we consider in Eqs. (4.1)–(4.4), is highly dependent on the cell population dynamics and interactions. For instance, let's consider the tumor cells. In solid cancers, they form heterogeneous populations with varying drug sensitivities that depend on multiple factors, such as the cell cycle stage [28], the presence of geno- or phenotype features [29], and the environmentally mediated drug resistance [30].

Under the antifragile control of drug dose, the tumor–immune–drug model is a dynamical system whose state space is not a vector space but rather a curved state manifold (i.e., the drug dose–response surface), more precisely a place and a dynamics to push the system towards [31].

For our therapy control problem, we want to push the tumor–immune–drug system to the desired dynamics of the drug dose-response surface, turning this into a tracking control problem. Recall that we want to have two attractor states lying on manifolds whose curvature (i.e., second derivative) is informative on the joint populations' dynamics.

In this study, the purpose of the antifragile controller is to drive the state $q(t) = [I(t), T(t), N(t), u(t)]^T$ of the tumor–immune–drug system toward a reference point on the desired/reference configuration $r(t)$—capturing the dynamics of the system in the antifragile region of the drug dose–response surface (see West et al. [16]). The first step in the controller design is the definition of a control error function, quantifying how far the system state is from the reference.

The control error function, $\varphi : Q \to \mathbb{R}$, describes the distance between the reference state (i.e., the tumor–immune–drug system dynamics in the antifragile region on the desired drug dose–response shape) denoted by r and the actual configuration/state q on a state manifold Q. In our case, the reference dynamics is determined by the position of the tumor–immune–drug system trajectory on the drug dose–response curve that describes the survival rate S versus drug dose u. Here, a lower survival is better as it accounts for more tumor kill and reaching the antifragile control region. In our case, we consider φ a uniformly quadratic function with constant L. This implies that, for all $\epsilon > 0$, there exist $b_1 \geq b_2 > 0$ such that

4.2 Closed-Loop Antifragility in Tumor-Immune-Drug Dynamics

$$b_2 \left\| \frac{d\varphi(q,r)}{dq} \right\|^2 \leq \varphi(q,r) \leq b_1 \left\| \frac{d\varphi(q,r)}{dq} \right\|^2 \tag{4.5}$$

In our case, we consider the configuration $q(t) = [I(t), T(t), N(t), u(t)]^T$ and the reference $r(t) = [I_S(t), T_S(t), N_s(t), u_S(t)]^T$. The control error φ is the most important component in ensuring the redundant overcompensation through its temporal evolution $\varphi(t)$ and its velocity $\dot{\varphi}(t)$.

4.2.4.1 Control Synthesis

In the current section, we formally introduce the three key components for antifragile control synthesis, namely redundant overcompensation, structure variability, and bounded high-frequency control activity.

Redundant overcompensation

We start the synthesis of the redundant overcompensation component which will induce the anticipation capabilities of the antifragile controller. From a control theoretic point of view, this accounts for a combined Proportional Derivative (PD) control action. Let's start with the more general form of our tumor–immune–drug model as a dynamical system in the Riemannian manifolds framework such as

$$\dot{q}(t) = v(t), t \geq 0 \tag{4.6}$$

$$\nabla_{\dot{q}} \dot{q} = \mathbb{S}(t, q(t), v(t)) + F(q(t)) \tag{4.7}$$

where q is the state, $\dot{q}$ is the velocity of the state, $\mathbb{S}$ is the time varying-state-transition map $\mathbb{S}: \mathbb{R} \times TQ \to TQ$, ∇ is the Riemannian covariant derivative, and F the control law.

As in the "traditional" PD control design, we need the error function between the state q (i.e. configuration) and the reference r, as well as the anticipation component. We consider the previously introduced error function φ on the manifold Q. The antifragile proportional gain K_φ is a smooth self-adjoint positive tensor filed on the manifold Q, and $K_q: T_qQ \to T_q^*Q$ is the antifragile derivative gain. Putting everything together, the antifragile PD control law for therapy design is computed as

$$F(q) = K_\varphi \varphi(q) + K_q \dot{\varphi}(q) \tag{4.8}$$

where $q(t) = [I(t), T(t), N(t), u(t)]^T$. This law is consistent with similar approaches for simple PD control on manifolds [38]. As a trademark of antifragile control, the first term in the Eq. (4.8), $K_q \dot{\varphi}(q)$, seeks to anticipate (not to predict) a higher level of error than the previous maximum through a redundant overcompensation that builds extra-capacity through the choice of the transport map that determines the term $K_q \dot{\varphi}(q)$. This component is responsible for driving the system closer the the desired dynamics, so we now evaluate the (Lyapunov) stability of the closed-loop given the control law $F(q)$.

Structure variability

While there are many advanced approaches, such as adaptation based on response identification and state observation or absolute stability techniques, the most straightforward way to deal with uncertainty is to keep certain limitations by "brute force". However, any carefully maintained equality eliminates one "uncertainty dimension". The theory of variable structure control (VSC) developed around this principle [39] and opened up a wide new area of development known as sliding mode control (SMC), that is characterized by a discontinuous control action which changes structure upon reaching a set of predetermined switching surfaces [40, 41]. The main advantages of using SMC in our therapy control design are listed below:

- the motion equation of the sliding mode [42] can be designed linear and homogeneous, despite that the tumor–immune–drug model is governed by nonlinear equations,
- the sliding surface does not depend on the process dynamics, but it is determined by parameters selected by the designer [43], i.e., desired trajectory of the system in the antifragile region of the drug dose–response curve (e.g., Hill function),
- once the sliding motion occurs (i.e., the system dynamics are on the surface), the system has invariant properties which make the motion independent of certain system parameter variations, uncertainty, and disturbances [44]. Hence, the system performance can be completely determined by the dynamics of the sliding manifold.

The first design element in the variable structure SMC is the choice of the sliding surface. Starting from the control error function φ, we define S as a time-varying surface in the state space/configuration space q, where

$$S(q, t) = \left(\frac{d}{dt} + \lambda\right)^{n-1} \varphi, \ \lambda > 0. \tag{4.9}$$

For instance, if $n = 2$ then $S(q, t) = \dot{\varphi} + \lambda\varphi$, if $n = 3$ then $S(q, t) = \ddot{\varphi} + 2\lambda\dot{\varphi} + \lambda^2\varphi$, and so on. As we see in Fig. 4.3b, the sliding surface is a curve in $(q, \dot{q})$ space of slope λ and containing the time-varying reference configuration $r(t)$. Recall that, for the "redundant overcompensation", the system follows the time-varying state transition $\mathbb{S}$. In SMC, the controller needs to "force" the system trajectories to "move" while still pointing towards the surface as depicted in Fig. 4.3a, b and theoretically proven in [42]. In other words, the curvature needs to decrease along the system trajectories such that

$$\frac{1}{2}\frac{d^2 S}{dt^2} \leq -\eta |S|, \ \eta > 0. \tag{4.10}$$

4.2 Closed-Loop Antifragility in Tumor-Immune-Drug Dynamics

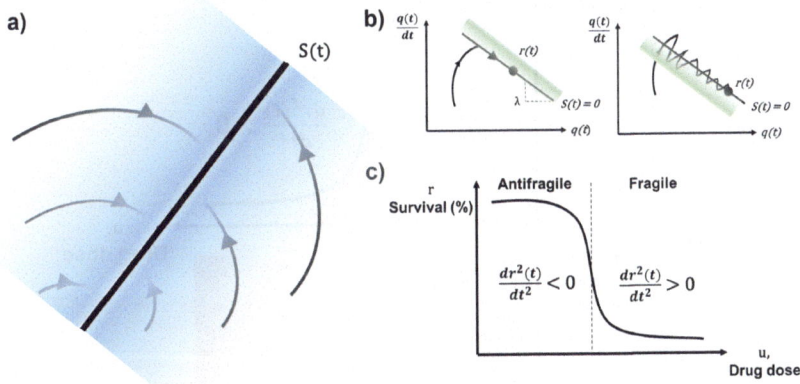

Fig. 4.3 Variable structure control using SMC. **a** the sliding condition, from initial states, the system is pushed towards the surface S; **b** the dynamics on the sliding surface; **c** drug dose–response curve with fragile and antifragile regimes depending on curvature (see West et al. [16])

The sliding condition in Eq. (4.10) makes the surface S an invariant set, which is both a place in the $(q, \dot{q})$ space as well as a dynamics that the system will follow once reaching the surface, i.e., when $\mathbb{S} = S$ (see Eq. (4.7)).

Particularized to antifragile therapy control, the desired configuration can be given by a vector $r(t)$ which will be "pushed", given the control law F to the convex (i.e.. antifragile) region of the drug dose–response depicted in Fig. 4.3c and mathematically described as

$$r = r_{min} + \frac{r_{max} - r_{min}}{1 + (\frac{u}{\mu})^{-n}}. \qquad (4.11)$$

For the definition of the survival in Eq. (4.11), we consider the Hill function with r_{min} minimal survival and r_{max} maximal survival, μ is the inflexion point of r beyond which increases of the drug have less impact on survival and n the Hill exponent. Note that the Hill function is a commonly employed mathematical model used to parameterize dose-response assays [45], although other functions might be used. In our experiments, we consider the parametrization in [16], where: $r_{min} = 20$, $r_{max} = 100$, $n = 10$, $\mu = 10$.

The reference state $r(t)$ (i.e., the configuration) is computed such that the dynamics of the tumor–immune–drug dynamics network model is driven to the antifragile region of the survival curve in Fig. 4.4a using an antifragile control law synthesized through the combined effect of the anticipation $K_q \dot{\varphi}(q)$ and the variable structure component $\beta \, \text{sgn}(S)$ of the controller, which ensure the curvature decrease along the system state trajectory (see the green region in Fig. 4.4b).

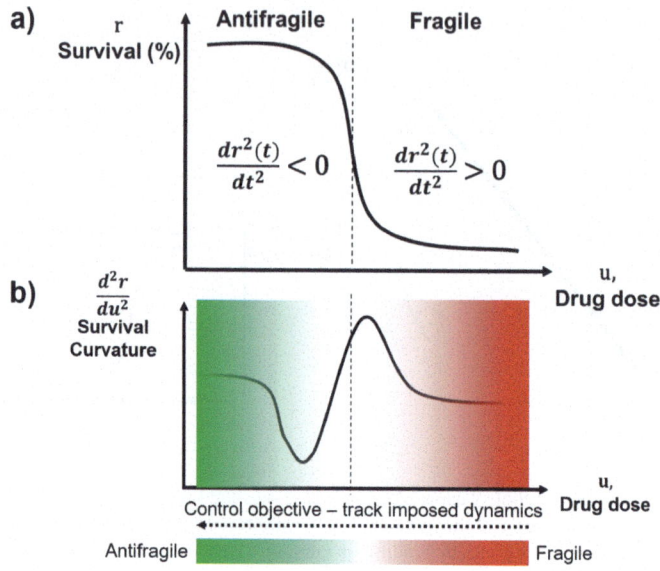

Fig. 4.4 Antifragile principle. **a** The drug dose–response basis for the imposed dynamics of the network. The survival function assumes that the system needs to provide a drug dose such that the value of r decreases; **b** The derivative of the survival function. This demonstrates that the inflexion point describes the point where the dosage (control law) can drive the tumor–immune–drug system in the antifragile region (see West et al. [16])

Putting all together, and hence combining the redundant overcompensation of the PD component in the antifragile design with the variable structure of the SMC, we have the following expression of the control law,

$$F(q) = K_\varphi \varphi(q) + K_q \dot{\varphi}(q) + \beta \, \text{sgn}(S), \tag{4.12}$$

where β is the SMC control gain and $\text{sgn}(S)$ is the sign function applied to the chosen sliding surface S, parametrized such that the condition in Eq. (4.10) is fulfilled.

4.2.5 State-of-The-Art Control Algorithms in Cancer Therapy

Control-theoretic therapy design is used to describe treatment protocols which have the potential to be more efficient (i.e., maximize tumor kill, minimize patient toxicity) than standard static periodic protocols now in use [48]. As discussed in the introduction, static therapy plans cannot cope with the highly nonlinear phenomena emerging in tumor–immune–drug network models, such as periodic oscillations in tumor and normal cells generation [17, 19], the resonance–antiresonance in drug response and toxicity [13, 20, 49], or the synchronization in tumor–environment cells interactions under drug pulses [?][21]. To handle such phenomena intrinsic in the tumor–immune–drug network, many control theoretic approaches were developed since the 80s, with notable work in [23, 51] and up to recent work in [52, 53].

4.2.5.1 Optimal Control

In the optimal control synthesis, the goal is to determine the therapy dose function $v(t)$ in Eq. (4.4), representing the chemotherapy administration schedule [23, 24, 56]. This is computed such that the kill rate of the tumor cell population is as high as possible, with the constraint that the killing rate of normal cells is minimized. Although for our experiments, we consider the simplified approach in [23], the general optimal control problem can be stated as follows.

The goal is to find the control variable, in our case, the therapy dose $v(t)$ in Eq. (4.4), and the (possibly free) final time t_f, corresponding to the end of therapy (e.g., after 150 days), that solves the following optimization problem

$$\begin{aligned} \underset{v, t_f}{\text{minimize}} \quad & J(v, t_f) = \varphi(x(t_f), t_f) \\ \text{subject to} \quad & \dot{x}(t) = f(x(t), v(t), t), \ t_0 \leq t \leq t_f, \\ & g(x(t)) \geq 0. \end{aligned} \quad (4.13)$$

In the optimization problem (4.13), the objective function $J = \varphi(x(t_f), t_f)$ is the tumor burden of the patient given the changes in the interacting cell populations N, T, I described by $x(t)$ and their evolution $f(x(t), v(t), t)$ under the drug administration. The state constraint $g(x(t))$ is used to maximize tumor kill and keep normal cells above a threshold. This formulation keeps the tumor cell population T lower at t_f at the price of large oscillations.

We update the problem such that we can weight each component of the objective function to avoid oscillations in the network model of Eqs. (4.1)–(4.4). We then rewrite the objective function J as a weighted combination of tumor burden at therapy end $T(t_f)$, the summed tumor burden over the treatment period $\int_0^{t_f} T(t)dt$, the maximum tumor burden over the treatment course $\max_{t \in t_o, t_f} T(t)$, and, of course, the drug dose concentration $u(t)$ during the therapy duration. The updated optimal control objective function J is given as

$$J(v, t_f) = w_1 T(t_f) + w_2 \int_0^{t_f} T(t)dt + w_3 \max_{t \in t_o, t_f} T(t) + w_4 u(t), \quad (4.14)$$

where w_i are weighting constants, chosen as $w_1 = 1500$, $w_2 = 150$, $w_3 = 1000$, $w_4 = 40$. To evaluate the effect the optimal control law has upon the tumor–immune–drug model, we plot the evolution of the system in Fig. 4.5.

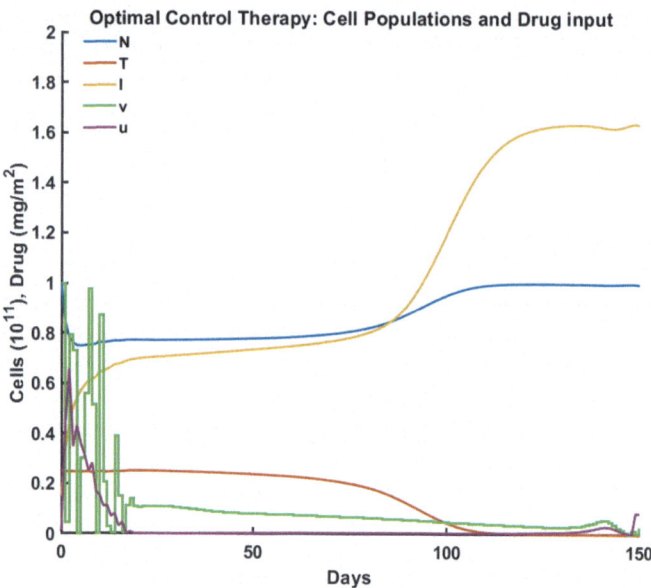

Fig. 4.5 Optimal control therapy. Individual cell populations evolve under optimal computation of the drug dose v. The drug dosing amplitude, timing, and duration are computed as a constrained optimization problem that slows down and, eventually, disrupts tumor growth. When the tumor (T) decays under the detectable size (≈ 80 days), the normal cell population (N) restarts the normal proliferation pattern, and immune reaction (I) is enhanced to support the complete tumor extinction

4.2.5.2 Robust Control

Another line of research, which goes beyond the optimal control landscape, is the variable structure control, such as bang-bang control [57]. This approach allows for seamless compensation of un-modelled dynamics in the tumor–immune–drug model and parametric uncertainties alike [58, 59]. Such models capture the dynamics of the phase field model of tumor growth [39, 40] and the regularities of the cell population states to control the phase of the drug concentration. In our study, we considered the model in [24] with parametrization considerations from [57].

In our therapy design problem, the control signal v is restricted to be between a lower and an upper bound of dosage $0 \leq v(t) \leq v_{max}$, as suggested by oncology guidelines. Additionally, in a special case of the optimal control in Problem 4.13, v switches from one extreme to the other (i.e., is strictly never in between the bounds). This is referred to as a bang-bang therapy solution, explored in both [24, 57]. To formulate the bang-bang control synthesis, we derive the control Hamiltonian[2] of

---

[2] Note that, for the therapy control design, we use the control Hamiltonian that describes the conditions for optimizing some scalar function, basically the Lagrangian concerning a control variable, and not the dynamics of the system itself.

4.2 Closed-Loop Antifragility in Tumor-Immune-Drug Dynamics

the optimal control problem (see Eqs. (4.15)) to identify the switching function of the system (i.e., ensuring that the drug entering the patient at time t is bounded).

$$H = \lambda_1 \left(\frac{dI}{dt}\right) + \lambda_2 \left(\frac{dT}{dt}\right) + \lambda_3 \left(\frac{dN}{dt}\right) + \lambda_4 \left(\frac{du}{dt}\right) + \eta, \quad (4.15)$$

where the functions λ_i satisfy the co-state variables equations

$$\frac{d\lambda_1}{dt} = -\lambda_1 \left(\frac{\rho T}{\alpha + T} - c_1 T - d_1 - a_1(1 - e^{-u})\right) + \lambda_2 c_2 T,$$

$$\frac{d\lambda_2}{dt} = -\lambda_1 \left(\frac{\rho \alpha I}{(\alpha + T)^2} - c_1 I\right) - \lambda_2(r_1 - 2r_1 b_1 T - c_2 I - c_3 N - a_2(1 - e^{-u})) + \lambda_3 c_4 N,$$

$$\frac{d\lambda_3}{dt} = \lambda_2 c_3 N - \lambda_3(r_2 - 2r_2 N^2 - c_4 T - a_3(1 - e^{-u})) - \eta(t),$$

$$\frac{d\lambda_4}{dt} = -e^{-u}(a_1 \lambda_1 I + a_2 \lambda_2 T + a_3 \lambda_3 N).$$

(4.16)

The η is chosen to ensure that the normal cells N are above 75% of the tumor-free normalized carrying capacity for this experiment such that

$$\eta(t) = \begin{cases} 1 & \text{if } N \leq 0.75, \\ 0 & \text{otherwise.} \end{cases} \quad (4.17)$$

We can now rewrite the robust control equation for the drug dosing as

$$\frac{\partial H}{\partial v} = \lambda_4, \quad (4.18)$$

which is independent of the control variable v. If we assume that the amount of drug entering the patient at time t is bounded above and satisfies $0 \leq v(t) \leq v_{max}$, then the output of the bang-bang control is given by

$$v(t) = \begin{cases} 0 & \text{if } \lambda_4 > 0, \\ v_{max} & \text{if } \lambda_4 < 0, \\ \text{singular} & \text{if } \lambda_4 = 0. \end{cases} \quad (4.19)$$

As we can see in Eq. (4.19), the co-state variable λ_4 is the switching function for the tumor–immune–drug network model we consider. In this case, the drug should be injected at the maximum rate when λ_4 is negative and should be ceased when λ_4 is positive. To evaluate the effect the robust control law has upon the tumor–immune–drug model, we plot the evolution of the system in Fig. 4.6.

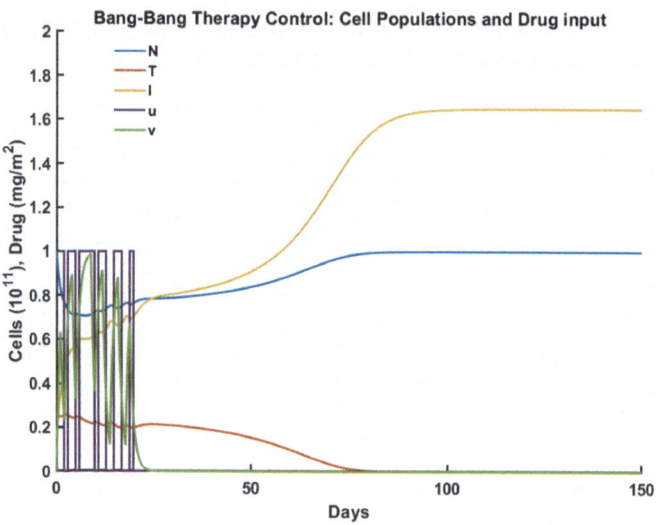

Fig. 4.6 Robust control therapy. Individual cell populations' evolution under the computation of the robust control law of drug dose v based on Eq. (4.16). The bang-bang drug dose timing and duration are computed such that the tumor population (T) decreases rapidly after treatment cessation (≈ 50 days). This decrease in tumor size is also determined by the exponentially increasing immune response (I) and marks the normal cell (N) proliferation/death (i.e., through toxicity) pattern

4.2.5.3 Pulsed Control

Pulsed control therapy assumes that the administration of the drug into the patient's body is modeled by a train of Dirac impulses. This approach is the traditional approach to chemotherapy and was approached by multiple studies [15, 60]. To parametrize the control system one needs to specify: (1) the total number of treatment sessions N (basically the total number of impulses); (2) the time interval between treatment sessions Tn (inter-impulse time interval); and (3) the drug dose administered in each session An (accounting for the amplitudes of the impulses).

Despite its simplicity, this control method is not applied in isolation [15]. The control variable v, represented by a train of Dirac impulses, is typically computed in the optimal control framework. Furthermore, the control design issue may be reduced to a finite-dimensional optimization problem that can be addressed by an appropriate solution, given that the control variable exerts a linear influence on the model and we adhere to an apriori established number of impulses. To evaluate the impact of the pulsed control law on the tumor-immune-drug model, the evolution of the system is plotted in Fig. 4.7.

In conclusion, the fundamental optimal impulsive control sequence is employed in a receding horizon strategy to generate a feedback control law. This strategy involves applying the initial control action of the sequence to the patient and repeating the

4.2 Closed-Loop Antifragility in Tumor-Immune-Drug Dynamics

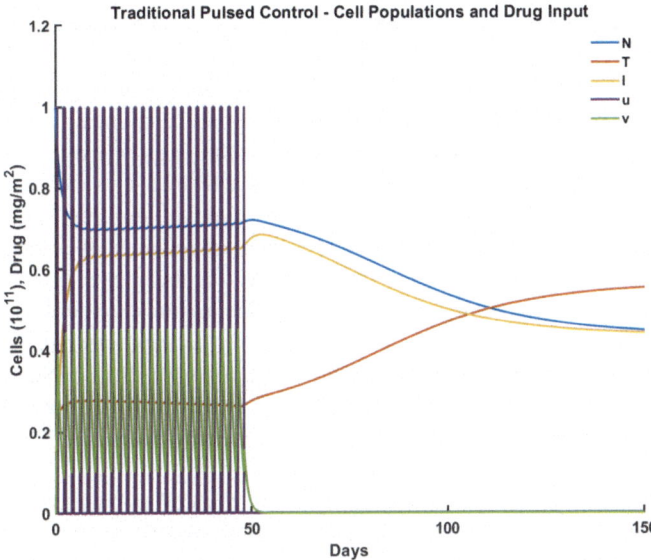

Fig. 4.7 Pulsed control therapy. Individual cell populations evolve under the computation of the robust control law of drug dose v. The pulsed control computes densely timed, equally sized, and dosed drug administrations, which only trigger short decays in tumor (T) proliferation, which at the end of the therapy resumes its uncontrolled growth, which suppresses the normal cells (N) production and a weakening immune response (I)

entire dynamic optimization process, commencing with the patient's state at the subsequent discrete time instant, as illustrated in [15].

4.2.5.4 Therapy Algorithmics

In clinical practice, it is typical to adhere to a defined treatment regimen wherein a consistent dosage is administered regularly. Notwithstanding, there are numerous instances wherein the tumor exhibits enhanced responsiveness to a 'volatile' treatment regimen in comparison to continuous therapy. A dose control strategy that is characterized by volatility (or as an "uneven" approach) has the potential to disrupt the tumor growth dynamics, leading to an instability that can be further accentuated by the joint action of the drug and the immune system and ultimately culminate in tumor elimination. Our experimental investigations, which employed asymmetric networks to elucidate the interactions between the tumor, the immune system and the drug, have shed light on these intriguing observations.

In our study, we were interested in exploring how antifragile control can offer a systematic approach to control drug dosage in "volatile" treatment plans where the drug "unevenness" can determine a fast tumor elimination with a good trade-off in drug quantity administration and collateral normal cell damage (i.e., toxicity induced cell death).

In consideration of the administration of the drug, the traditional pulsed approach is distinguished by the lowest maximum drug concentration among all methods. This is accompanied by the limitation that the impact on tumor growth dynamics is only marginal, and this begins to diverge once the regimen reaches its maximum delivery program. The remaining methods result in a higher maximum drug concentration, reaching up to 80% more, but with the advantage of reducing the tumor burden throughout between 65 and 80 days. It is noteworthy that the most efficient approach in terms of drug quantity is the robust control, which administered only 12 mg/L of the drug during therapy. However, due to its delivery pattern, specifically in terms of frequency and timing, it reached the highest maximum drug concentration of 0.987 mg/L. The antifragile control method employed a moderate total drug dose of 14.31 mg/L, distributed over the entire 150-day therapy period, with a maximum dose of 0.736 mg/L.

In consideration of the individual evolution of the cell populations within the tumor-immune-drug model, it can be observed that the pulsed therapy is the treatment which resulted in the largest tumor size of 0.553×10^{11} cells at day 150 of the therapy regimen. This is attributed to the limited delivery schedule and the conservative dosage employed. This also results in the inefficiency of tumor elimination and, of course, a high loss in the preservation of normal cells, many of which were killed due to the high toxicity level. This is evidenced by the considerable loss of normal cells, amounting to 0.447×10^{11} cells after the therapeutic regimen. Conversely, the antifragile control exhibited the greatest efficacy in tumor eradication, with the robust and optimal control approaches demonstrating comparable outcomes. This is, of course, motivated by the weighted objective functions in the case of optimal and robust controllers and the advantages of anticipation and high-frequency control activity of the antifragile control. With a minimal tumor burden of 0.251×10^{11}, the antifragile controller elicited sustained, high-frequency control activity for the entire duration of the therapy, but with moderate drug administration and concentration.

Ultimately, when evaluating the impact of therapy on normal cells, as quantified by the minimum number of normal cells, the optimal control emerges as the most effective, with a maximum of 0.750×10^{11} cells, followed by the robust and antifragile approaches. Overall, the antifragile control demonstrates a rapid reduction in tumor burden, even with moderate drug administration and concentration, while achieving the highest tumor kill and moderate collateral damage to normal cells through drug-induced toxicity.

4.2.6 Interventional Antifragility in Clinical Practice

An emerging approach used to leverage second-order effects to mitigate the evolution of treatment resistance in cancer is known as adaptive therapy [1]. In a recent clinical trial (NCT02415621) in metastatic castrate-resistant prostate cancer. Rather than

4.2 Closed-Loop Antifragility in Tumor-Immune-Drug Dynamics

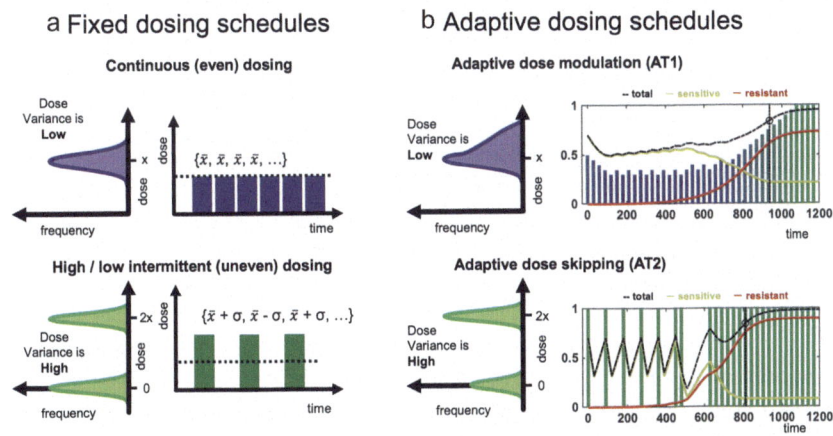

Fig. 4.8 a Example fixed dosing schedules where schedules are determined apriori for fixed, prescribed doses given at periodic and regular intervals. Schedules range from continuous (even) schedules associated with low variance (purple) to intermittent schedules with a high degree of variance. **b** An alternative to fixed dosing is known as adaptive dosing, where the dose prescribed is determined based on the response of a patient-specific biomarker, which may rise or fall at each decision time point. Algorithms for dosing range from dose modulation (top), which is typically associated with low variance, or dose skipping, associated with high variance

follow the standard-of-care regular intervals of identical doses (see Fig. 4.8a), this trial introduced irregular dosing that was determined by an algorithm based on the tumor's response (see Fig. 4.8b). Treatment was initiated until a biomarker response (a proxy for tumor size) of 50% decline was obtained, and treatment was paused until the biomarker level returned to 100% of the original value. The justification for this approach was to maintain a sufficient tumor burden with ostensible treatment-sensitive cells that inhibit the growth of resistant cells. The group hypothesized the existence of a cost of resistance, whereby resistant cells divide less rapidly than cells without costly mechanisms of resistance [1–3]. These adaptive algorithms lead to a decrease in the cumulative dose administered to a patient [4, 5].

Mathematical modeling integrated with preclinical or clinical data has spurred the development of improved algorithms to drive dosing [6–11]. Two main algorithms are proposed: adaptive dose modulation (see Fig. 4.8b, top) and adaptive dose skipping (see Fig. 4.8b, bottom). As seen in the figure, each algorithm has an emergent mean and distribution of dosing that is time-dependent (and patient-specific). More research is required to optimize both first-order and second-order effects for patient benefit.

4.3 Closed-Loop Control of Epilepsy

4.3.1 Problem Statement

Another disease that can be understood from an antifragility perspective is epilepsy. Epilepsy is one of the most common neurological disorders, with a prevalence of almost 1% in the general population [62]. It is a brain disorder that can be characterized by the predisposition to occurrences of unprovoked seizures. Although various treatments and medications exist, these fail to achieve seizure control in around a third of patients.

Bionic solutions have been successful in cases where medication is not suitable. Open-loop stimulation and deep-brain stimulation devices have also significantly improved conditions in many cases. However, due to the invasive nature of these technologies, complications can occur from scar tissue formation and surgery-related problems. Hence, it is important to maximize the lifetime of these implants. Indeed, the lifetime of implants is currently one decade.

In contrast to open-loop stimulation, closed-loop stimulation takes neural activity into account. Hence, it can, in principle, be driven by biomarkers, rendering it advantageous concerning efficiency and battery life. Nevertheless, closed-loop stimulation technologies also require implants that can exert strong stimulation, which can entail the usage of multiple implants. Despite significant improvements in implant technology and associated biocompatibility, such responsive neurostimulation implants are not (yet) used in regular clinical practice. However, initial clinical trials indicate a promising impact, and important steps towards its real-world application have been accomplished [66, 67].

It remains an open question of how to best program the closed-loop stimulation protocols to minimize implant surgery while delivering effective seizure control. We propose that mathematical techniques that conceptualize the epileptic brain, somewhat counterintuitively, as an anti-fragile system, could lead to a quantitative framework to optimize responsive neurostimulation. Improvement of epileptic conditions through a personalized external control of closed-loop stimulation could be realized by leveraging the knowledge of the condition's approximated antifragile behavior. We here describe relevant factors that need to be considered when designing such an anti-fragile controller.

Antifragile systems are associated with convex response dynamics [65]. As such, epilepsy can be understood as an antifragile condition of the brain: seizures can occur without external stimulation, i.e., patients can suffer from seizures at times when there is no obvious trigger. Additionally, it is well-established that certain types of stimulation can evoke seizures, such as, for instance, certain high-frequency visual signals. Figure 4.9 shows graphically the convexity of epilepsy.

Given that epilepsy can be understood as an antifragile system, the challenge is to develop therapies and interventions that are also antifragile. Much more, they should be able to out-compete the epileptic convexity. Given that every brain is different, the question becomes more complex, as the exact shape and dynamics

4.3 Closed-Loop Control of Epilepsy

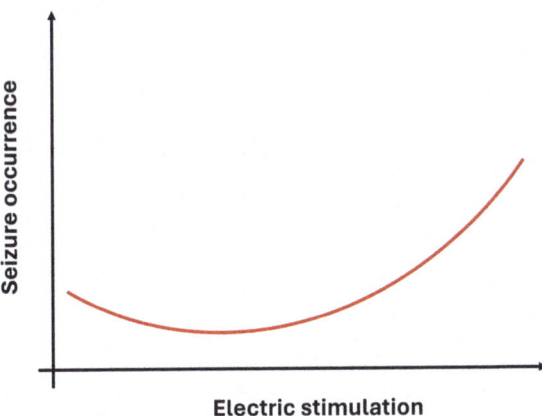

Fig. 4.9 Illustration of convexity in epilepsy. Epilepsy can be understood as an antifragile phenomenon due to the convexity in its response to stimulation. An epileptic patient who receives no stimulation will usually experience seizures even without notable causes from the external environment, e.g. during sleep. On the other hand, significant stimulation patterns, such as visual stimulation at certain frequencies, can further increase the frequency of seizure activity. In the middle region, controlled intervention, e.g., from implants, can often ameliorate the condition. It is this sweet spot where therapeutic intervention can contribute significantly to clinical impact

of the antifragile behavior will vary significantly, due to the highly heterogeneous nature of the disorder. Hence, personalized approaches are paramount for realistic therapies, as explained in the cancer-related treatment above.

4.3.2 Personalization of Therapeutic Intervention in Epilepsy

The human brain comprises almost 100 billion neurons, each with approximately 10,000 chemical synapses. Each neuron has some slight individualities, be it concerning its morphology, distribution of receptors or gene expression. No two brains are identical. This raises the question of how to adjust interventions for a given patient. Computational methods are necessary here due to the vast amount of data that needs to be accounted for. It is beyond the scope of this book to give a comprehensive overview of relevant work, and the interested reader is recommended the following recent works [63, 64].

References

1. Robert A Gatenby, Ariosto S Silva, Robert J Gillies, and B Roy Frieden. Adaptive therapy. *Cancer research*, 69(11):4894–4903, 2009.
2. Jeffrey West, Yongqian Ma, and Paul K Newton. Capitalizing on competition: An evolutionary model of competitive release in metastatic castration resistant prostate cancer treatment. *Journal of Theoretical Biology*, 455:249–260, 2018.
3. Robert A Gatenby. A change of strategy in the war on cancer. *Nature*, 459(7246):508, 2009.
4. Jingsong Zhang, Jessica J Cunningham, Joel S Brown, and Robert A Gatenby. Integrating evolutionary dynamics into treatment of metastatic castrate-resistant prostate cancer. *Nature Communications*, 8(1):1816, 2017.
5. Jingsong Zhang, Jessica Cunningham, Joel Brown, and Robert Gatenby. Evolution-based mathematical models significantly prolong response to abiraterone in metastatic castrate-resistant prostate cancer and identify strategies to further improve outcomes. *Elife*, 11:e76284, 2022.
6. Jeffrey West, Fred Adler, Jill Gallaher, Maximilian Strobl, Renee Brady-Nicholls, Joel Brown, Mark Roberson-Tessi, Eunjung Kim, Robert Noble, Yannick Viossat, David Basanta, and Alexander RA Anderson. A survey of open questions in adaptive therapy: Bridging mathematics and clinical translation. *eLife*, 12, March 2023.
7. Jill A. Gallaher, Pedro M. Enriquez-Navas, Kimberly A. Luddy, Robert A. Gatenby, and Alexander R.A. Anderson. Spatial heterogeneity and evolutionary dynamics modulate time to recurrence in continuous and adaptive cancer therapies. *Cancer Research*, 78(8):2127–2139, April 2018.
8. Maximilian A.R. Strobl, Jeffrey West, Yannick Viossat, Mehdi Damaghi, Mark Robertson-Tessi, Joel S. Brown, Robert A. Gatenby, Philip K. Maini, and Alexander R.A. Anderson. Turnover modulates the need for a cost of resistance in adaptive therapy. *Cancer Research*, 81(4):1135–1147, February 2021.
9. Maximilian A. R. Strobl, Jill Gallaher, Jeffrey West, Mark Robertson-Tessi, Philip K. Maini, and Alexander R. A. Anderson. Spatial structure impacts adaptive therapy by shaping intra-tumoral competition. *Communications Medicine*, 2(1), April 2022.
10. Jeffrey West, Li You, Jingsong Zhang, Robert A Gatenby, Joel S Brown, Paul K Newton, and Alexander RA Anderson. Towards multidrug adaptive therapy. *Cancer research*, 80(7):1578–1589, 2020.
11. Jeffrey B. West, Mina N. Dinh, Joel S. Brown, Jingsong Zhang, Alexander R. Anderson, and Robert A. Gatenby. Multidrug cancer therapy in metastatic castrate-resistant prostate cancer: An evolution-based strategy. *Clinical Cancer Research*, 25(14):4413–4421, 2019.
12. Nia, H.T.; Munn, L.L.; Jain, R.K. Physical traits of cancer. *Science* **2020**, *370*, eaaz0868.
13. Schättler, H.; Ledzewicz, U. Optimal control for mathematical models of cancer therapies. *An application of geometric methods* **2015**.
14. Kurz, D.; Sánchez, C.S.; Axenie, C. Data-driven Discovery of Mathematical and Physical Relations in Oncology Data using Human-understandable Machine Learning. *Frontiers in Artificial Intelligence* **2021**, *4*.
15. Belfo, J.P.; Lemos, J.M. *Optimal Impulsive Control for Cancer Therapy*; Springer, 2020.
16. West, J.; Strobl, M.; Armagost, C.; Miles, R.; Marusyk, A.; Anderson, A.R. Antifragile therapy. *bioRxiv* **2020**.
17. Kim, M.; Gillies, R.J.; Rejniak, K.A. Current advances in mathematical modeling of anti-cancer drug penetration into tumor tissues. *Frontiers in oncology* **2013**, p. 278.
18. McDonald, E..; El-Deiry, W.S. Cell cycle control as a basis for cancer drug development. *International journal of oncology* **2000**, *16*, 871–957.
19. Hu, X.; Jang, S.R.J. Dynamics of tumor–CD4+–cytokine–host cells interactions with treatments. *Applied Mathematics and Computation* **2018**, *321*, 700–720.
20. Agur, Z.; Kheifetz, Y. Resonance and anti-resonance: from mathematical theory to clinical cancer treatment design. *Handbook of Cancer Models with Applications to Cancer Screening, Cancer Treatment and Risk Assessment* **2005**.

References

21. Agur, Z.; Kheifetz, Y. Optimizing Cancer Chemotherapy: From Mathematical Theories to Clinical Treatment. In *New Challenges for Cancer Systems Biomedicine*; Springer, 2012; pp. 285–299.
22. Pillis, L.d.; Radunskaya, A. Modeling Immune-Mediated Tumor Growth and Treatment. In *Mathematical Oncology 2013*; Springer, 2014; pp. 199–235.
23. De Pillis, L.G.; Radunskaya, A. The dynamics of an optimally controlled tumor model: A case study. *Mathematical and computer modelling* **2003**, *37*, 1221–1244.
24. De Pillis, L.G.; Radunskaya, A. A mathematical tumor model with immune resistance and drug therapy: an optimal control approach. *Computational and Mathematical Methods in Medicine* **2001**, *3*, 79–100.
25. Taleb, N.N. *Antifragile: Things that gain from disorder*; Vol. 3, Random House, 2012.
26. Taleb, N.N. (anti) fragility and convex responses in medicine. International Conference on Complex Systems. Springer, 2018, pp. 299–325.
27. Goutelle, S.; Maurin, M.; Rougier, F.; Barbaut, X.; Bourguignon, L.; Ducher, M.; Maire, P. The Hill equation: a review of its capabilities in pharmacological modelling. *Fundamental & clinical pharmacology* **2008**, *22*, 633–648.
28. Gaffney, E.A. The application of mathematical modelling to aspects of adjuvant chemotherapy scheduling. *Journal of mathematical biology* **2004**, *48*, 375–422.
29. Fedorinov, D.S.; Lyadov, V.K.; Sychev, D.A. Genotype-based chemotherapy for patients with gastrointestinal tumors: focus on oxaliplatin, irinotecan, and fluoropyrimidines. *Drug Metabolism and Personalized Therapy* **2021**.
30. Paraiso, K.H.; Smalley, K.S. Fibroblast-mediated drug resistance in cancer. *Biochemical pharmacology* **2013**, *85*, 1033–1041.
31. Bejenaru, A.; Udriste, C. Riemannian optimal control. *arXiv preprint* arXiv:1203.3655 **2012**.
32. Lee, J.M. *Riemannian manifolds: an introduction to curvature*; Vol. 176, Springer Science & Business Media, 2006.
33. Bloch, A.M. An introduction to aspects of geometric control theory. In *Nonholonomic mechanics and control*; Springer, 2015; pp. 199–233.
34. Zou, L.; Wen, X.; Karimi, H.R.; Shi, Y. The identification of convex function on Riemannian manifold. *Mathematical Problems in Engineering* **2014**, *2014*.
35. Bullo, F.; Murray, R.M. Proportional derivative (PD) control on the Euclidean group. *Caltech Reports* **1995**.
36. Bécigneul, G.; Ganea, O.E. Riemannian adaptive optimization methods. *arXiv preprint* arXiv:1810.00760 **2018**.
37. Fiori, S. Manifold Calculus in System Theory and Control—Fundamentals and First-Order Systems. *Symmetry* **2021**, *13*, 2092.
38. Fiori, S.; Cervigni, I.; Ippoliti, M.; Menotta, C. Synchronization of dynamical systems on Riemannian manifolds by an extended PID-type control theory: Numerical evaluation. *Discrete and Continuous Dynamical Systems-B* **2022**.
39. Guo, Y.; Xu, B.; Zhang, R. Terminal sliding mode control of mems gyroscopes with finite-time learning. *IEEE Transactions on Neural Networks and Learning Systems* **2020**, *32*, 4490–4498.
40. Colli, P.; Gilardi, G.; Marinoschi, G.; Rocca, E. Sliding mode control for a phase field system related to tumor growth. *Applied Mathematics & Optimization* **2019**, *79*, 647–670.
41. Ouyang, P.; Acob, J.; Pano, V. PD with sliding mode control for trajectory tracking. *Robotics and Computer-Integrated Manufacturing* **2014**, *30*, 189–200.
42. Slotine, J.J.E.; Li, W.; others. *Applied nonlinear control*; Vol. 199, Prentice hall Englewood Cliffs, NJ, 1991.
43. DeCarlo, R.A.; Zak, S.H.; Matthews, G.P. Variable structure control of nonlinear multivariable systems: a tutorial. *Proceedings of the IEEE* **1988**, *76*, 212–232.
44. Utkin, V. Variable structure systems with sliding modes. *IEEE Transactions on Automatic control* **1977**, *22*, 212–222.
45. Meyer, C.T.; Wooten, D.J.; Paudel, B.B.; Bauer, J.; Hardeman, K.N.; Westover, D.; Lovly, C.M.; Harris, L.A.; Tyson, D.R.; Quaranta, V. Quantifying drug combination synergy along potency and efficacy axes. *Cell systems* **2019**, *8*, 97–108.

46. Maithripala, D.S.; Berg, J.M. An intrinsic PID controller for mechanical systems on Lie groups. *Automatica* **2015**, *54*, 189–200.
47. Zhang, Z.; Sarlette, A.; Ling, Z. Integral control on Lie groups. *Systems & Control Letters* **2015**, *80*, 9–15.
48. Lecca, P. Control Theory and Cancer Chemotherapy: How They Interact. *Frontiers in Bioengineering and Biotechnology* **2021**, *8*, 621269.
49. Li, D.; Xu, W.; Guo, Y.; Xu, Y. Fluctuations induced extinction and stochastic resonance effect in a model of tumor growth with periodic treatment. *Physics Letters A* **2011**, *375*, 886–890.
50. Ren, H.P.; Yang, Y.; Baptista, M.S.; Grebogi, C. Tumour chemotherapy strategy based on impulse control theory. *Philosophical Transactions of the Royal Society A: Mathematical, Physical and Engineering Sciences* **2017**, *375*, 20160221.
51. Swan, G.W. Role of optimal control theory in cancer chemotherapy. *Mathematical biosciences* **1990**, *101*, 237–284.
52. Carrere, C. Optimization of an in vitro chemotherapy to avoid resistant tumours. *Journal of Theoretical Biology* **2017**, *413*, 24–33.
53. Irurzun-Arana, I.; Janda, A.; Ardanza-Trevijano, S.; Trocóniz, I.F. Optimal dynamic control approach in a multi-objective therapeutic scenario: Application to drug delivery in the treatment of prostate cancer. *PLOS Computational Biology* **2018**, *14*, 1–16.
54. Uthamacumaran, A. A review of dynamical systems approaches for the detection of chaotic attractors in cancer networks. *Patterns* **2021**, *2*, 100226.
55. Axenie, C.; Kurz, D. Chimera: Combining mechanistic models and machine learning for personalized chemotherapy and surgery sequencing in breast cancer. International Symposium on Mathematical and Computational Oncology. Springer, 2020, pp. 13–24.
56. Wang, S. Optimal control for cancer chemotherapy under tumor heterogeneity. 2019 IEEE 58th Conference on Decision and Control (CDC). IEEE, 2019, pp. 5936–5941.
57. Ledzewicz, U.; Maurer, H.; Schättler, H. Bang-bang and singular controls in a mathematical model for combined anti-angiogenic and chemotherapy treatments. Proceedings of the 48h IEEE Conference on Decision and Control (CDC) held jointly with 2009 28th Chinese Control Conference. IEEE, 2009, pp. 2280–2285.
58. Ledzewicz, U.; Schättler, H. Optimal bang-bang controls for a two-compartment model in cancer chemotherapy. *Journal of optimization theory and applications* **2002**, *114*, 609–637.
59. Ledzewicz, U.; Schättler, H.; Gahrooi, M.R.; Dehkordi, S.M. On the MTD paradigm and optimal control for multi-drug cancer chemotherapy. *Mathematical Biosciences & Engineering* **2013**, *10*, 803.
60. Panetta, J.C. A mathematical model of periodically pulsed chemotherapy: tumor recurrence and metastasis in a competitive environment. *Bulletin of mathematical Biology* **1996**, *58*, 425–447.
61. Kelly, M. An Introduction to Trajectory Optimization: How to do your own Direct Collocation. *SIAM Review* **2017**, *59*, 849–904.
62. Beghi, E. The epidemiology of epilepsy. *Neuroepidemiology*. **54**, 185–191 (2020).
63. Jirsa, V., Wang, H., Triebkorn, P., Hashemi, M., Jha, J., Gonzalez-Martinez, J., Guye, M., Makhalova, J. & Bartolomei, F. Personalised virtual brain models in epilepsy. *The Lancet Neurology*. **22**, 443–454 (2023).
64. Singh, K., Osswald, M., Ziesenitz, V., Awchi, M., Usemann, J., Imbach, L., Kohler, M., Garcia-Gomez, D., Anker, J., Frey, U. & Others Personalised therapeutic management of epileptic patients guided by pathway-driven breath metabolomics. *Communications Medicine*. **1**, 21 (2021).
65. Taleb, N. & West, J. Working with convex responses: Antifragility from finance to oncology. *Entropy*. **25**, 343 (2023).
66. Turnbull, M., Hazra, A., Gandara, C., McLeod, F., McDermott, E., Escobedo-Cousin, E., Idil, A., Bailey, R. & Others Closed-loop optogenetic control of the dynamics of neural activity in non-human primates. *Nature Biomedical Engineering*. **7**, 559–575 (2023).
67. Ghosh, S., Sinha, J., Ghosh, S., Sharma, H., Bhaskar, R. & Narayanan, K. A comprehensive review of emerging trends and innovative therapies in epilepsy management. *Brain Sciences*. **13**, 1305 (2023).

Chapter 5
Conclusions

Abstract This chapter concludes our interdisciplinary endeavor into natural systems antifragility. Be it ecological, evolutionary, or interventional, antifragility expands and consolidates the typical analysis and modelling of natural systems. We hereby offer the main concepts that define antifragility levels in natural systems as well as the new research avenues our insights offer.

5.1 Ecological (Anti)-Fragility

Ecologically antifragile systems benefit from the inhomogeneity of the internal dynamics distribution based on the convexity of the system's response function without external input and solely based on the heterogeneity and resilience of the internal components. This describes, in other words, the function of the system without external input, based solely on the heterogeneity and resilience of the internal components. Characteristics such as stability describe the simplest system response with minimal antifragile properties. Within this scale, the precise characterization of the payoff function, which represents the relationship between system inputs and outputs, is paramount.

In biological systems, changes in environmental conditions can reduce the survival and fecundity of individuals based on a species' Darwinian fitness. The rate of change of environmental perturbations can reduce fitness in response to stochastic fluctuations and seasonal variations. The payoff function associated with the system's response to environmental variation can be concave (fragile), convex (antifragile), or linear (neutral) [4].

Ecological antifragility is the natural system counterpart to intrinsic antifragility and can be defined as the system benefit derived from input volatility. The definition of ecological fragility or antifragility is useful for predicting and managing a biological population. For example, mathematical models describing the response to anticancer drugs measure the ecological effect of volatile versus continuous treatment schedules, with or without drug pharmacokinetics.

Neural processing is another very good study case that offers a complex system that recapitulates a large repertoire of dynamics. Neural networks must maintain their stability under perturbations on timescales ranging from milliseconds to months or even years. It seems paradoxical, but neural networks can only remain stable if they are excitable and able to adapt their response (and structure) in response to external stimuli. Changes in neuronal excitability regulate the functionality of neural networks by absorbing a wide range of molecular and cellular parameter changes while maintaining their spiking functionality. For example, homeostatic activity regulation in single neurons enables resilience to recurrent state variable changes, which correlates with resilience to parameter changes due to the critical slowing phenomenon.

Similar to technical systems, criticality in natural systems is related to antifragility. Empirical studies have suggested that living systems operate close to critical thresholds that exist on the delicate boundary between order and randomness, as demonstrated in various domains, including electrical heart activity and brain function. Accurate measurement of the payoff function plays a key role in predicting antifragility to the scale of planetary ecosystem antifragility by integrating well-established principles from non-equilibrium thermodynamics and adopting a system dynamics approach using Fisher's information on Earth's entropy production [5].

In summary, antifragility can be quantified by a geometric analysis of the shape of the nonlinearity characterizing the payoff function. It is important to note that antifragility is a scale measure of the effect of variation at the level of statistical singularities (divergence of the high-order statistical moments). Here, depending on the type of system (natural or technical), the assessment of antifragility is tied to the measure of the benefit (or harm) of input distribution irregularities, volatility or disturbances due to the nonlinearity of the system's payoff function.

5.2 Evolutionary (Anti)-Fragility

Homogeneity and heterogeneity play a crucial role in the design and synthesis of inherited and evolutionary antifragile systems. From criticality and multi-level interactions of multiple timescales to the quantification of criticality margins, such a design scheme exploits local interactions of the system to interactions of the system to make it benefit from perturbations. In other words, evolutionary antifragile systems benefit from the unevenness of the input distribution based on the emergent system dynamics and its interactions with the operating environment (i.e., noise, modulated perturbations).

Evolution, defined here as the change in heritable traits within a population over time, is also influenced by environmental perturbations. Ecological antifragility considers individual species in isolation to quantify the response to perturbation. Evolutionary antifragility quantifies how a heterogeneous population of interacting species is affected by perturbations. For example, in cancer, competition between heterogeneous populations of cell types modulates antifragility. In biological systems, we study complexity (which implies maximum computational capacity) and how systems reach criticality. The adaptive mechanisms of living systems must not only respond to environmental variability through random mutation followed by selection but must also have built-in properties that allow them to discover alternatives to adapt to adversity, variability and uncertainty. Using theoretical arguments, it has been proposed that systems undergoing eco-evolution tend to be at criticality, which implies maximum complexity and inference capacity, and then they are also at maximum antifragility. Stability plays a central role in the functioning of both natural and technical dynamical systems. Paradoxically, a dynamical system can only remain stable if it is excitable and able to change its behavior in response to external stimuli. It is flexible and, therefore, stable; in fact, the true stability of the organism depends on its modest instability. Inherited antifragility in natural systems is a consequence of interactions between all components through evolutionary processes (e.g. genetic inheritance, microbiome inheritance and social inheritance) constrained by external conditions. Antifragile natural systems arise under uncertainty, stress and perturbation at both ecological and evolutionary scales [6]. Evolution by natural selection itself can be thought of as an antifragile process, where a population is maintained by genetic variation in the face of environmental perturbations. For example, although individuals within a population may die, the population evolves towards a more antifragile state with increasingly higher fitness to cope with fluctuating environmental conditions.

In that sense, just as in thermodynamically isolated systems where the arrow of entropy points to the most probable outcome of a thermodynamic process, it seems to us that in complex adaptive systems, there is an equivalent arrow of antifragility. This arrow indicates that after a perturbation and the system's subsequent adaptation to it, from a set of possible future scenarios, the system will evolve toward the most antifragile one, consistent with the system's context. If this turns out to be true, then the antifragility concept would be as foundational to complex systems as entropy to thermodynamic systems [7].

5.3 Interventional (Anti)-Fragility

Inducing desired behavior within interventional antifragility requires an innovative, control-theoretic design and synthesis approach. Here, non-linear dynamics in space and time can promote the system's ability to absorb internal and external perturbations. Interventional antifragile systems benefit from uneven input distribution based on emergent system dynamics in closed-loop control with a controller to drive the system towards a prescribed dynamic in the presence of modulated or transient disturbances, noise and volatility.

Designing intervention strategies to eradicate a heterogeneous population can be extremely difficult due to the evolution of resistance to interventional treatments. For example, continuous administration of anticancer drugs or antibiotics selects for resistant subpopulations, rendering subsequent treatments ineffective. Recent work applying principles from agricultural methods, known as integrative pest management, has shown some success in cancer treatment. For example, adaptive cancer therapy uses a simple rule-of-thumb protocol to adjust treatment administration and break intervals based on tumor response [3]. Importantly, this adaptive protocol results in an increase in dose variance (prolonged periods of high dose followed by prolonged periods of zero dose). This is part of a broader effort to use evolutionary principles to design treatment protocols that increase the treatment-induced volatility that tumor cells undergo during treatment to maximize tumor regression. Mathematical models of tumor-immune-drug interactions can guide the optimization of chemotherapy regimens to maximize the efficacy/toxicity ratio [2].

In addition, several recent papers have shown that dietary patterns may influence network communication along the brain-gut axis, especially at the age when both systems are undergoing maturation processes. From an ecological perspective, an adequate level of From an ecological perspective, adequate levels of connectivity mitigate the effects of perturbations in species distributions and increase ecosystem stability. A loss of connectivity leads to a loss of antifragility in the gut microbiota ecosystem. The basic idea is that a system's response to perturbations requires an efficient flow of information. For maximum antifragility, this flow must be optimal, which implies maximum connectivity.

References

1. Axenie, C., López-Corona, O., Makridis, M., Akbarzadeh, M., Saveriano, M., Stancu, A. & West, J. Antifragility in complex dynamical systems. *Npj Complexity*. **1**, 12 (2024).
2. Axenie, C., Kurz, D. & Saveriano, M. Antifragile Control Systems: The Case of an Anti-Symmetric Network Model of the Tumor-Immune-Drug Interactions. *Symmetry*. **14**, 2034 (2022,10), https://www.mdpi.com/2073-8994/14/10/2034, Number: 10 Publisher: Multidisciplinary Digital Publishing Institute.
3. Nassim Nicholas Taleb and Jeffrey West. Working with convex responses: Antifragility from finance to oncology. *Entropy*, 25(2):343, February 2023.
4. López-Corona, O., Kolb, M., Ramírez-Carrillo, E., Lovett, J. (2022). ESD Ideas: planetary antifragility: a new dimension in the definition of the safe operating space for humanity. Earth System Dynamics, 13(3), 1145–1155.
5. López-Corona, O., & Padilla, P. (2019). Fisher information as a unifying concept for criticality and antifragility: A primer hypothesis. ResearchersOne. https://doi.org/10.13140/RG.2.2.28789.73444
6. Jeffrey West, Jill Gallaher, Maximilian Strobl, Mark Robertson-Tessi, and Alexander R.A. Anderson. The fundamentals of evolutionary therapy in cancer. In *Cancer Systems Biology and Translational Mathematical Oncology*. Oxford University Press, 2023.
7. López-Corona, O., Ramírez-Carrillo, E., and Magallanes, G. (2019). The rise of the technobionts: toward a new ontology to understand current planetary crisis. *Researchers.One*. https://researchers.one/articles/19.01.00001v1

The manufacturer's authorised representative in the EU is Springer Nature Customer Service Centre GmbH, Europaplatz 3, 69115 Heidelberg, Germany. If you have any concerns regarding our products, please contact ProductSafety@springernature.com

Printed and bound by CPI Group (UK) Ltd, Croydon, CR0 4YY

26/03/2026

02078972-0005